DR. CHRISTINE LE

AUTISM RULES

HOW TO THRIVE
IN A NEURODIVERSE WORLD

Autism Rules: How to Thrive in a Neurodiverse World
Copyright © 2022 by Christine Le

Thank you for purchasing an authorized edition of this book and for complying with copyright laws by not reproducing, scanning, or distributing any part of it in any form without permission.

ISBN: 9798835153886

The information contained in this book is for educational purposes only and is not intended to be a substitute for professional medical advice, diagnosis, or treatment.

*For Ian, Ralph
and
all who have taught me.*

Thank you.

CONTENTS

	Introduction	7
Chapter 1	Preliminary Rules	13
Chapter 2	Consciously Learn the Unwritten Rules	23
Chapter 3	Strengthen Your Social Radar	55
Chapter 4	Educate Others About How Your Mind Works	109
Chapter 5	Celebrate Your Differences and if People Don't Like It, Too Bad for Them	131
Chapter 6	The Rules Checklist	175
Chapter 7	Resources	181
Chapter 8	References	189

INTRODUCTION

It was 1999, I had just finished my doctorate in psychology and had started to specialize in autism, and I had a lot of questions and few answers. Why did the six-year-old with autism throw my Lego block on the floor every time I tried to add it to his castle? Why was the teenager refusing to write a paragraph about the weekend she had enjoyed at the beach? My clients on the spectrum approached things differently and I appreciated their rich and complex thinking, but if I was going to be of any help it was clear that I needed to build more bridges between their world and mine.

I knew that to find the answers was going to require research, so I attended conferences, read books, went to trainings, and had guidance from other therapists. I accompanied my clients to their daily classes, to occupational therapy, speech therapy, to their homes, community, and work sites. I attended IEP meetings, developed goals and interventions, took data, wrote reports, counseled families, and diagnosed people from age five to seventy. But most of all I listened. I listened to what people had to say about their own experiences. It was like stepping into another culture and trying my best to understand.

Gradually patterns began to emerge, rules of thinking that helped me understand. For instance, I learned that people with autism often have a specific way that they want to create something and that other people's additions can be viewed as "wrong." I also discovered that it can be hard for someone on the spectrum to translate visual memories of a weekend into words on a page. I am now at a point in my profession and in working with my clients where my answers are more than my questions. When clients come in with their challenges, I usually have suggestions as to how to resolve them. Some of these challenges have immediate solutions. One young boy Aiden was having frequent tantrums about choosing clothes for school. When it was cold he would want to wear shorts, when it was hot he would put a sweater on. His parents encouraged him to pick out his clothes the night before, but then he would change his mind at the last moment. Mornings in the house had become so stressful that it had begun to affect his parents' work. Aiden was very interested in the weather, but the problem with words such as "cold" and "hot" is that they are abstract; it's like saying to someone "be nice." For a concrete thinker like Aiden, it was confusing.

After exploring this in the session, Aiden and his parents worked on a solution that was concrete—a chart with different temperature ranges and the appropriate clothing he could wear. We made sure that he was involved in writing the temperatures down and drawing pictures of the clothes. This would be his chart. Each day he would look at what temperature it was going to be at twelve pm and choose his clothes accordingly. It was a simple solution that was immediately effective as it respected certain rules of helping autistic people—be aware of concrete thinking, integrate areas of interest (the weather), provide space for the person to be involved in developing a solution, and start with the assumption that the person is not intentionally being oppositional.

For others, change is more gradual. Rachel was already in college when she came to see me. She was a talented math student who had struggled throughout her life with anxiety, depression, opposition, and thoughts of suicide. She had been in therapy several times and received different diagnoses including oppositional defiant disorder (ODD), generalized anxiety disorder (GAD), and depression. While it was true that she had met the criteria for each of these, it seemed that the most important piece of information had been missed – the possibility that she had undiagnosed autism. We spent the first few sessions completing an assessment which confirmed that she was on the spectrum. Rachel was both surprised and confused; it was something she had never considered.

Introduction

However, it was after she received her diagnosis that the crucial part of our work began. It involved looking back at her experiences through the framework of autism. We discovered that her behavior that was assumed to be oppositional, such as leaving a family gathering early, was not due to Rachel being disrespectful, but was a response to sensory overload. The noise from all the talking and music hurt her ears, the lights of the house were too bright. When she didn't look her family in the eyes, they assumed she was being rude, but the eye contact made it hard for her to focus on what others were saying. Rachel had tried to socialize, but these attempts often ended poorly, heightening her anxiety the next time she talked to people. She stressed about saying the wrong thing and making people angry. It's understandable how this spiraled down into withdrawal, depression, and thoughts of "I'm a bad person" or "I shouldn't be here."

As we worked, self-hatred slowly began to be replaced with self-compassion, and she made small changes to acknowledge her past achievements and strengths. For example, instead of thinking that her anxiety made her weak, she saw how continuing to try to talk to people had required an incredible strength. She acknowledged that going through middle school, high school, and college with her unique challenges was an achievement. She had succeeded despite the fact that she had so much more to manage than other people, such as continuously analyzing the words that people were using in their sentences in order to figure out their emotions. Rachel had assumed everyone did this, but that she just wasn't as good at it as others. With the new understanding of her mind, Rachel started to make sense of her world.

I find that my clients experience a certain freedom in discovering who they are and how their minds work, and their families and friends become hopeful that there are solutions to the challenges. I am always excited to see a client who has just tried a new intervention because what I usually hear is, "This stuff really works."

"Yes," I'll reply. "It does."

It was an adult client on the spectrum who told me that I should write this book. "I was struggling for years until you helped me understand my mind," he said one day. "There are others out there who need this information." So here

Introduction

we are—I've compiled over 20 years of insight into a practical, straightforward guide to help a neurodiverse person and their family and friends, not just survive, but thrive in a neurotypical world.

This book is organized into sections of rules and it is written to the person who is on the spectrum. If you are on the spectrum, you will find that rules are useful. They are concrete, clear and can be used across the lifespan. If you are not on the spectrum, but you are reading this book because you have a child, friend, or family member who is, the rules will give you guidelines for understanding and helping the person on the spectrum.

Chapter 1 outlines rules on how social information is processed, and why it is that being different can lead to so many challenges. Unspoken social rules are everywhere, and if your social radar is not picking up or sending out information in the same way as others, you can end up being misunderstood.

In working with numerous people with autism, I have learned to recognize which challenges are the most common. For example, many people struggle with talking too long about an area of interest or with trying to answer a question both honestly and kindly. The rules in Chapter 2 cover all of the common challenges. If you learn and practice them, you will be well-prepared to cope with many of the difficulties in your life.

Chapter 3 has rules addressing how to strengthen your social skills. In a world where your social interactions can determine everything from being employed to having friends, it is important that you become as good as you can at your social interactions.

Chapter 4 outlines the traits of an autistic mind. As your mind works differently from others, it's important to understand what these differences are, how to educate others about how your mind works, and how to use the differences as a strength. I have written these traits in a list so that you or your family can check off the ones that apply to you. There are also strategies for managing challenges associated with each specific trait. I have tried to make the list practical, easy to use, and relevant for all ages.

Chapter 5 is my favorite because it has rules about celebrating who you are. There are many talented people with a mind like yours. They are often

Introduction

kind, dedicated, and direct. They are people whose greatest strength is to see things differently and who have the courage to change the world.

Lastly, in Chapter 6, you will find a checklist where all the rules in the book are compiled and briefly listed. Here you can check off the rules you have mastered and note the ones you want to set as goals. And in Chapter 7, you will find a list of resources and how to reach out to them for additional support.

Throughout the book you will see cartoons that are aimed at giving a humorous look at some of our social constructs. To highlight the voices of people on the spectrum there are quotes from different autistic people written in italics. Any specific details of clients such as age, gender, or circumstances have been altered to protect their identity.

The language that I use in the book is aimed at helping people to feel empowered when talking about autism. Some of my clients prefer person-first language such as "a person with autism." They feel this language helps to emphasize their humanity. Others prefer identity-first language such as "autistic person." This recognizes autism as an important part of their identity. As a therapist wanting to support all people on the autism spectrum and their diversity of perspectives, I will be using both people-first and identity-first language. If you have any preference, I encourage you to communicate it to the people in your life, while supporting others on the spectrum who feel differently.

As a psychologist I always have the goal of making my clients the experts. I want them to learn everything that I have learned—to have the tools that I have. I want them to not need me.

It is my sincerest wish that this book will help in this endeavor.

CHAPTER 1

Preliminary Rules

When I ask my clients who are on the spectrum if they feel different from others, the majority say "yes." Some have felt different since the age of five. Others say that they feel as though they "come from another planet." In this chapter we will explore how social information is processed and why it is that being different can lead to so many challenges.

BEING DIFFERENT IS NOT THE SAME AS BEING WRONG

The reality is that if you have been diagnosed with an Autism Spectrum Disorder (ASD), then you are different. You might think differently, act differently, process emotions differently. You probably know it, and many people around you know it too. But being different is not the same as being wrong.

The equation $2 + 1 = 4$ is wrong. We look at the number 4 and know that it shouldn't be there. We want to replace it with a 3. However, $2 \neq 1$ is correct and makes no judgment about the numbers on either side of the equation. They are just different, not wrong.

So why is autism even considered a problem, especially for those people who are higher functioning? The only reason is that you are in the minority. If autistic people had the majority, tags on clothing would be outlawed, colleges would drop the requirement to take a wide range of subjects, and I would be in therapy because I would keep looking people in the eyes and making them feel uncomfortable.

MOST SOCIAL RULES ARE UNWRITTEN

Imagine everyone you know is a bird and you just happen to be a bug or a fish.

Unwritten social rules are everywhere. And I mean everywhere. For many of you they begin to raise their ugly heads somewhere around 4th grade. At this stage social rules become more complicated than, "Do you want to be my friend?" and what is seen as a cute behavior in kindergarten might now be viewed as annoying.

For someone on the spectrum, this can be a particularly sad and frustrating time. It is often pre-diagnosis and it's hard to understand why things aren't working out as they used to. You might not know that unwritten rules exist or that you are breaking them. Clients describe how they get up in the morning with their hearts full of hope that today will be different, today they will make a friend or play with the group, only to discover that their efforts are rejected.

When this happens day after day, week after week, month after month, the rejection from others can turn to self-loathing and feeling vulnerable and disconnected. I'll often hear children who are going through this say, "I hate myself," "I'm stupid," or "I should have never been born."

So why is it that breaking social rules leads to rejection? And how it is that everyone knows the rules and you don't?

Preliminary Rules

IF YOU BREAK AN UNWRITTEN SOCIAL RULE, PEOPLE WILL BECOME ANGRY OR ANXIOUS AND MAKE A JUDGMENT ABOUT YOU WHICH IS USUALLY NEGATIVE AND WRONG

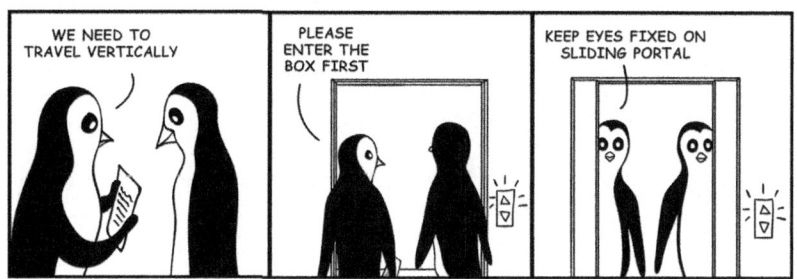

To help people understand the impact of breaking an unwritten social rule, I'll ask them to do the "Elevator Experiment." Imagine that you are inside an elevator. You look around, and see a lot of written rules inside. There are notices on the wall like "in case of emergency press button," or "maximum weight 3,000 pounds." But elevators also have a lot of invisible rules that are difficult to detect. One of these rules is, "When standing in an elevator you must face the door."

To do the "Elevator Experiment" pick a building with an elevator where you are not likely to see people you know. Get in the elevator and stand with your back to the door. You will be facing everyone and everyone else will be facing you. This gives you the perfect position to study people's reactions as you break the unwritten rule. You will probably see a lot of anxiety (shifting feet, eyes looking down, people moving away from you) and even anger (angry challenging stares). This is what happens when you break unwritten rules. It makes people uncomfortable, anxious, and angry.

As you break the unwritten rule, everyone else will try to make sense of your behavior. They will wonder, "Why is this person facing the wrong way? What's wrong with them?" As people don't like the ambiguity of not knowing, they will eventually come to some sort of judgment. Sadly, it's usually not a correct one. Few people will wonder, "Is this person on the autism spectrum and he doesn't know he is breaking an unwritten rule?" They are more likely to make one of the judgments listed below.

When you break the elevator rule:

Other people may feel	Uncomfortable Anxious Angry
People Make a Judgment They may think you are . . .	Challenging them Drunk or on drugs Threatening

Whether it's the elevator rule, or the breaking of a friendship rule in fourth grade, when others feel uncomfortable and make negative judgments about you, they are more likely to reject you. They will move away from you, stop talking to you, and not want to be your friend.

THE TYPICAL PERSON NAVIGATING SOCIAL RULES IS LIKE A BAT NAVIGATING WITH ECHOLOCATION

When bats fly in the dark they make a high pitch sound that sends out sound waves. These waves hit objects in the environment, and echo waves travel back to the bat.

The bat's brain processes the information in the echo waves to form an understanding of the things around it. It will know the size of an object and the distance and movement of objects close to it. The bat can then make changes in its position to avoid obstacles and other animals. This system of navigation is called echolocation.

Preliminary Rules

A neurotypical person (someone not on the autism spectrum) also has a radar—The "Social Radar." As the person moves around, she is constantly sending out social waves such as a smile, body position, or vocalization. These waves travel out to a second person, and the second person sends back an echo wave with information. The echo wave might be a smile, a frown, or a subtle body movement. The first person's brain interprets all the information in the echo wave, and she will adjust her behavior depending on what she wants. The adjusted behavior becomes a new social wave which is sent out.

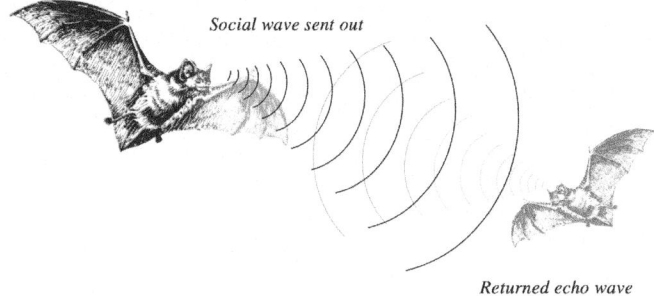

Social wave sent out

Returned echo wave

Social Wave Sent Out
▼
Returned Echo Wave
▼
Interpretation of the Echo Wave
▼
**Adjusted Behavior /
New Social Wave Sent Out**

The following two examples show how this might work if you are standing in line at a supermarket. Each example has a different adjusted behavior.

A man has just cut in front of you . . .

SOCIAL WAVE SENT OUT	RETURNED ECHO WAVE	INTERPRETATION OF THE ECHO WAVE	ADJUSTED BEHAVIOR / NEW SOCIAL WAVE SENT OUT
You step forward in line, getting closer to the man who has just cut in front of you.	The man who has just cut in front of you moves two steps forward, their hand goes up to the back of their neck, and they turn their head slightly towards you.	The man feels uncomfortable with you standing so close.	You move back again. You don't want the man to feel uncomfortable from you standing too close.
You step forward in line, getting closer to the man who has just cut in front of you.	The man who has just cut in front of you moves two steps forward, their hand goes up to the back of their neck, and they turn their head slightly towards you.	The man feels uncomfortable with you standing so close.	You stay where you are. You want the man to know that he shouldn't have cut in front of you.

This social radar is going on constantly and is mostly unconscious. It is a continual process of sending out social waves, receiving the returned echo wave, interpreting the returned echo wave, and adjusting behavior.

Preliminary Rules

It is unheard, unspoken, and can pick up the smallest pieces of information, such as someone slightly clenching his hand or a subtle change in a tone of voice. It can process social waves from a whole room of people or from one person sitting alone.

The social radar also has the ability to store and remember information. It can learn information in one situation, store it in the brain, and have it ready to use in another situation. Your typical person doesn't even know it exists. It's something he doesn't usually have to think about; it all happens automatically.

To help typical people understand how automatic this process is, I'll sometimes ask, "How did you know what distance to stand from me as we came into my office?"

"I have no idea," they say with a confused look on their faces. "I've never really thought about it."

"Or what about if you walk into a movie theatre, and there's only one couple sitting in there. Would you know how many seats away you would need to sit so they don't feel uncomfortable?"

"Well yes, I'd know."

"How do you know? Did anyone ever tell you?"

"No, no one has."

And this is when they realize they know so many unwritten social rules they have never had to consciously learn. Their social radars have been up and running for years.

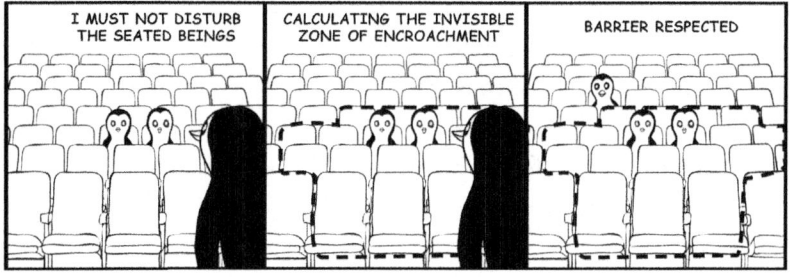

PEOPLE ON THE SPECTRUM HAVE A DIFFERENT SOCIAL RADAR

*I want to connect with people, I just
don't know how to do it.*

Being on the autism spectrum, you will have a different social radar. The first difference is that you may be sending out fewer social waves. You might find yourself using fewer facial expressions and gestures such as not using your hands as much to express yourself or nodding and shrugging less. Your tone of voice can be monotone. In other words, you are giving out a restricted range of social waves. The waves are not as varied, which makes it harder for others to know what you are thinking and feeling.

The second difference is that you can have difficulty understanding people's echo waves, and as a result you make fewer adjustments to your behavior. Reading the waves that come back from others is an important part of the social radar, but it can be challenging. You might fail to notice the subtle cues of another person or misinterpret them. There is a notion in the autism literature called "Mind Blindness." This term describes the idea that autistic people have difficulty reading other people's minds. In situations where a typical person makes a good guess at what someone else is thinking and feeling, the person on the spectrum struggles.

In sessions where family members are present, I'll sometimes ask the client on the spectrum, "What do you think your mom (or dad, wife, sister, brother, etc.) is thinking and feeling right now?" This is usually followed by a silence and then a guess, which is often wrong. What is interesting about the wrong guess is that it's usually based on what the client is thinking or feeling in that moment. If she is feeling angry, then it's "My mom's feeling angry." If she is feeling sad, "My brother's sad." The logic is that if that if she is feeling something, then the other person must be feeling it too.

Some autistic people have also described that it's difficult to read echo waves because of how much information their brains are receiving. They notice the sound of a ticking clock, the itchy feel of their jeans, the traffic outside

Preliminary Rules

the window, a mark from a coffee spill on the carpet, a paint chip, and small changes in the room such as a pillow in a different place or a new plant. With so much information coming in, it's understandable how reading another person's echo waves gets lost in all the noise. It would be like trying to watch a television show with several televisions playing different channels in the same room at the same time.

Again, please remember that this is not wrong. Your radar is not broken; it's just different. But to function in a world full of "bats," you have four things you can do:

1. Consciously learn the unwritten rules.
2. Strengthen your social radar.
3. Educate others about how your mind works.
4. Celebrate your differences and if people don't like it, too bad for them.

This book will cover all four approaches. I would encourage you to learn them all. There will be times in your life when you will need them.

AUTISM RULES

CHAPTER 2

Consciously Learn
The Unwritten Rules

In this chapter I break down the social rules that my clients on the spectrum struggle with the most including rules about hygiene, communication, honesty, party etiquette, caring for others and boundaries.

These rules are unwritten, and because it can be difficult to realize that they even exist, they are too often the cause of misunderstandings, broken relationships, and lost opportunities. For example, children on the spectrum are frequently isolated in the classroom because they correct their peers, and many adults lose friendships when they try to give an honest answer to a question or they talk too long about a subject they are interested in. However, when you consciously learn the unwritten rules, you can strengthen your relationships and thrive.

If you've already mastered a rule, then just skip over it. But for some people, missing one basic rule can be a deal-breaker. I've sat with people who have done everything right to get employment—gone to college, developed language skills, practiced social situations—and no-one will hire them. Sometimes it's simply because they need to wash their hair.

Too often I will hear a client say they wish someone had explained one of these rules to them so that they could have avoided a conflict or stressful situation.

HYGIENE

TAKE A SHOWER AND WASH YOUR HAIR EVERY DAY	Although statistics vary, we know that most Americans shower once a day. Use soap and shampoo. Rinse well.
USE DEODORANT EVERY DAY	If you smell bad, people will avoid you.
KEEP YOUR NAILS CUT AND CLEAN	If people see that your nails are dirty, they will assume that your overall hygiene is poor.
DON'T WEAR THE SAME CLOTHES TWO DAYS IN A ROW	Don't show up to work in what you wore the day before.

Consciously Learn The Unwritten Rules

COMMUNICATION

WHEN TALKING TO ANOTHER PERSON, SPEND MORE TIME TALKING ABOUT THAT PERSON'S INTERESTS THAN YOURS

This social rule is one of the most important but is also one that is often broken by people on the spectrum. It's not that others don't admire your passion and knowledge about your specific area of interest (they do), it's just that after a while they find it boring. Not everyone wants to know all the details.

Learning this rule can help in so many areas of your life: getting through an interview; going on a date; relationships with your parents, siblings, children, and spouse. It's a rule that just shouldn't be ignored. To know how to do this successfully, just follow the communication rules below.

BE AWARE THAT THE MAJORITY OF CONVERSATIONS ARE VERY SUPERFICIAL

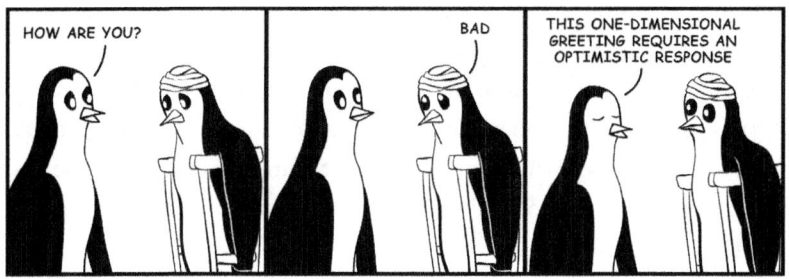

Be encouraged by the fact that most conversations are superficial. Superficial = easier to learn.

DEVELOP AN INDEX CARD IN YOUR MIND FOR EACH PERSON YOU INTERACT WITH ON A REGULAR BASIS

Talking to people feels like a game and I'm always losing. There's a strategy to it, and I don't know what it is.

People don't realize they have an index card system in their minds, but they use it all the time. When they see someone they know, an index card will be pulled up in their minds. It will have the other person's name along with information that is relevant to them.

For example, Catherine sees Jim at work and remembers that two days ago she had a conversation with him about his daughter's upcoming birthday party. Then without thinking much about it, she will say, "Hey Jim, how's it going?"

"Good."

"How was Sarah's party?"

Jim is now feeling great that someone remembered his daughter Sarah, and off he goes talking all about the bouncy castle.

One of the great strengths of being autistic is often a strong visual memory, so for this rule, you're going to use it to your advantage. If you don't have this strength, you can put notes in your phone or use actual cards. Just don't let anyone see them unless they are a family member, friend, or teacher who is helping you with your social skills.

At the top of the card visualize the person's name and his or her face next to the name. Then underneath the name, visualize the person's interests, activities, and observations you make about him. To discover these, listen carefully to what the person talks about. Categorizing the different areas that people talk about will help you.

Areas include:

Upcoming events—Vacations, trips, sporting events, kids' recitals.
Life changes—Moving, getting married, births, death.
Struggles—Sickness, financial, conflict, unemployment.

Family—Children, partner, parents, pets.
Memberships—Church, clubs, organizations.
Specific Interests—How does he spend his time?

USE THE 5WS

The majority of things going through my head are completely irrelevant to the conversation.

If you listen carefully to other people's conversations, you'll notice that the 5Ws come up a lot. These are the Who, What, Where, When and Why questions.

Remember that for now you're not trying to develop deep conversations on one topic. There will be time for this later—in the Celebrate your Differences chapter you will see how one man with autism, Satoshi Tajiri, formed a closer community for a subject he was particularly interested in. But for now, we are focusing on how to have good reciprocal communication. This is the back and forth chitchat of everyday life.

Listen carefully to other people and notice how they use the 5Ws. Examples include:

Who	Who were they playing? Who's teaching the class? That's a great idea. Who thought of it?
What	What was it like? What are you doing over the summer?
Where	Where did you work before here? Where did you get it?
When	When do you start your new job? When are you going?
Why	Why did you stop playing soccer? Why did you move?

COMBINE THE 5WS WITH YOUR INDEX CARD

Humans talk and talk and talk,
and I don't know what to say.

Now the next time you see a familiar-looking person visualize his index card with their name, interests, and activities. Pick a subject from the card, for example, "new job." Then run through the 5Ws in your mind, and match a question to the subject. For example, "What."

Casually ask your question, and then listen carefully to the answer. "What's your new job like?"

Some of what the person is saying will become new information that you can add to the index card. For example, "I have a presentation I need to give on Friday." Make a note of this under upcoming events.

Be aware that if you are at a special event such as a wedding, graduation, orientation at work, product promotion, or athletic event, keep your opening conversation related to the special event. This is because at that moment the person will usually be more interested in the special event, than other things in his life. You don't want to walk up to someone at a wedding and the first thing you say is, "How was Sarah's birthday party?"

This process is exactly what people do daily without thinking about it, the only difference is that for you it will be conscious. When you first start practicing, choose people you are most comfortable with. Some people start at home during a casual time such as dinner, using actual note cards in front of them. One set of cards can have the W questions, the other will have the names of family members with their interests. The more you practice, the easier it will become. Then you can move on to more challenging situations.

If you are a parent of a child with autism, this is a wonderful activity to do with your child.

IT'S USUALLY MORE IMPORTANT TO BE KIND THAN TO BE RIGHT

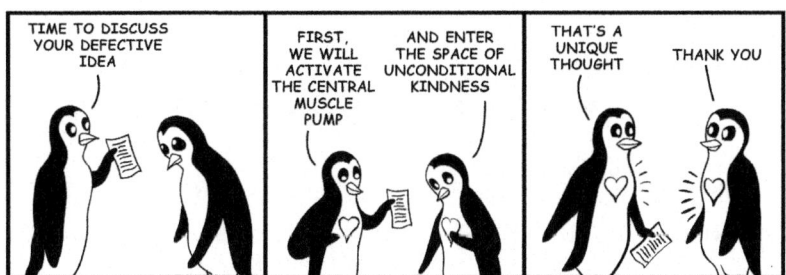

Many of you are very smart, but that can bring its own difficulties. Some people describe how hard it is sitting in class listening to students ask the same questions over and over. Others note how frustrated they become when someone insists that something is true, when it's clearly false. If your IQ is on the upper end of the scale or you have a good attention to detail, you'll notice the mistakes that others make. You'll see what should be fixed, how to do things better, but you'll also notice that not everyone appreciates your ideas (did you ever try pointing out your teacher's or boss' errors?). When you do speak up people will call you self-righteous, when you don't they'll think you're selfish or smug. So, what's a detail-orientated person on the spectrum supposed to do?

When you find yourself getting pulled into an argument, defending a point of view, or feeling angry due to someone's stupidity, remember the rule about being kind.

Kindness is not about saying, "You're right," when you know someone is wrong, but about helping the other person feel good about talking to you. It's about opening up communication, recognizing that there is more than one way to look at things, and realizing that another person may be trying his best. If a person is being kind to you, you need to be kind to him. Look at the following examples and see if you can relate them to any situations in your own life.

Imagine you are doing something and it starts to go wrong. You become annoyed, and Andrew steps in to help. He makes it worse. Now you're getting angry.

	WHAT YOU DO	HOW ANDREW FEELS
BEING RIGHT	You think about how incompetent and unhelpful Andrew is. You start to put him down.	Andrew is angry and thinking, "What an ungrateful ... I'm never going to help again."
BEING KIND	You think about how Andrew tried to help. You kindly direct him as to how he can help you best. "It would be great if you could ..."	Andrew is feeling good about being able to help. It's something he doesn't get to do too often as you're very independent and smart.

You're involved in a group project at school or work. Eleanor comes up with a really bad idea. The group seems to like it.

	WHAT YOU DO	HOW YOUR CLASSMATES FEEL	HOW OTHER WORKERS FEEL
BEING RIGHT	You tell Eleanor why it's a bad idea. You start to argue as Eleanor tries to defend herself in front of the group. She is humiliated and hating you right now.	If you're at school, some kids feel annoyed and make a note not to have you in their group next time. Others are afraid to speak up.	If you're at work, the boss thinks that you're difficult. He knows you're smart, but he's wondering if you're worth keeping around.

BEING KIND	You start by saying one thing you like. As you can't think of anything specific you use a general phrase such as "That's original," or "Yes, I can picture that." You then state your difficulty with it as an observation or a question. "I'm wondering what the cost of this will be?"	Your classmates feel relieved that you asked about the cost before it became a problem. Everyone starts to share their ideas on how it can be done cheaply.	Your work colleagues feel grateful to have you as part of the team. They think about how helpful and smart you are.

You're meeting Connor for the first time. Perhaps he's a fellow student, co-worker, or your daughter's new boyfriend. He starts to talk about your area of interest. Most of what he's saying is wrong.

	WHAT YOU DO	HOW CONNOR FEELS
BEING RIGHT	You correct Connor. He feels embarrassed and starts to argue back. It turns into a nasty debate.	The other people in the room feel very uncomfortable. Everyone is looking at you as being the problem, not Connor, who had all his facts wrong.
BEING KIND	You remember the kind rule. You lean forward and say to Connor, "That's interesting; I've never heard that before."	Your friends and family have a new appreciation for you.

THERE IS A COST TO FREE SPEECH

Never have there been so many opportunities for your thoughts and opinions to be heard. Thanks to social media, you can send your pictures and words around the world in a matter of seconds, and they can remain there for years. This may seem like a wonderful opportunity for your right to free speech until the party picture you posted in college stops you from getting your dream job when you graduate.

People have failed interviews, been fired, and even been jailed for things they have posted. Remember that private posts often go public. Remember that your words or images can cost you a job, relationship, client, and can ruin a good reputation in a matter of seconds.

Avoid posts that involve drinking, drugs, nudity, sexual content, hate comments, insulting words like "stupid" and "idiot," put-downs, politics, racism, rants, frustrations, and health issues (employers are not legally allowed to discriminate due to health issues, but it does happen).

HONESTY

PEOPLE WANT HONESTY, BUT THEY ALSO DON'T WANT TO BE HURT EMOTIONALLY

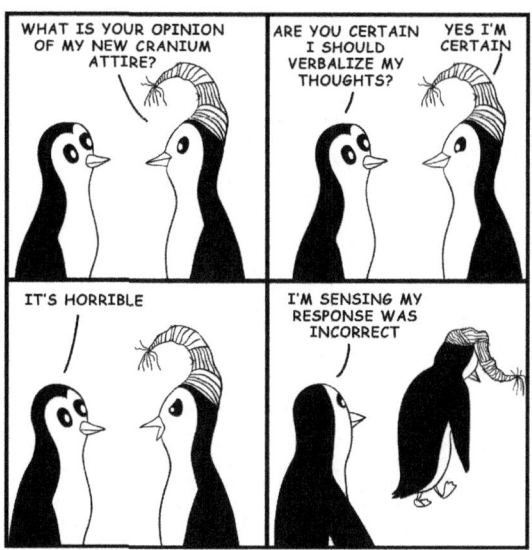

One of the great characteristics of many autistic people is their honesty. There is often a "what you see is what you get" quality to them. When you want an honest opinion, ask someone on the spectrum and she is likely to give you an honest answer. But the problem is that when people ask a question, they don't want your answer to make them feel bad. What is an honest person supposed to do? Lie?

Some people will say that "Everyone tells lies," and that a "little white lie" or a "good lie" is just fine. The problem with telling lies is that it usually leads to more difficulties and more lies. This can be especially challenging. You tell a lie to get out of a difficult social situation, only to find yourself in an even more challenging one. I don't believe that lies are ever needed, but you do need to learn how to answer a question honestly. Look at the flow chart as we go over the rules for answering difficult questions.

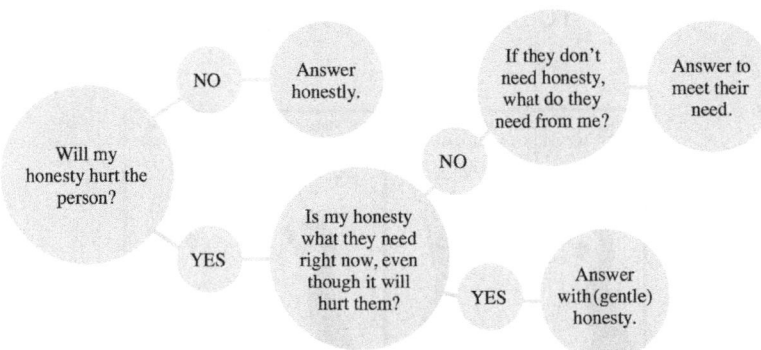

The first question to ask yourself is, "Will my honesty hurt the person?" When someone asks you a question, she wants an answer, but she also doesn't want to feel sad or discouraged.

You can learn to recognize when someone is feeling hurt. Study her face and body movements. Things to look for include looking down or away, not smiling, speaking softly, talking less, slumped posture, shrugging, tears, watery eyes, or moving away from you. Pay special attention to the things a person says more than once. People will often repeat things that are important to them but that you might have failed to understand or acknowledge. "But I thought you'd like to take this hat fishing," and "The hat's the same color as your fishing rod," is a repeat. She is trying to tell you she is excited about buying you this hat for your fishing.

Learn what types of answers are more likely to be hurtful such as:

—Telling someone he is not good at something (his recital was boring, dinner was disgusting, he made lots of mistakes in his computer program, he failed a test, the gift he chose for you is ugly).

—Giving someone bad news (dead pet or relative, he is sick, someone he knows is sick, the company is closing, you're breaking up with the person).

—Crushing dreams (he won't make the team or be the next CEO, you changed your mind about the camping trip with him).

—Telling someone he looks bad (clothes look bad, he looks old, the haircut is awful).

ANSWERS THAT DO NOT HURT A PERSON SHOULD ALWAYS BE GIVEN HONESTLY

If the answer to a question you have been asked is a simple, factual statement that will not hurt the person emotionally, go ahead and answer honestly. For example, someone asks you which restaurant you prefer or what ideas you have for an upcoming project at work. These answers should be given directly and honestly.

ANSWERS THAT WILL HURT THE PERSON, BUT ARE IMPORTANT FOR THE PERSON TO KNOW, SHOULD BE GIVEN WITH (GENTLE) HONESTY

When you ask me for the truth I'll give you the unfiltered, undiluted, unadulterated truth.

There will be many times in your life when you need to give someone information, and you know that it will make him or her feel bad. Life is messy, and you can't always protect others from the pain it brings. For example, you may need to tell someone that her cat is dead, you want to break up the engagement, or a person has three months to live. They need the information. You need to tell them.

There is a difference between brutal honesty and gentle honesty. In brutal honesty, the answer is given directly and quickly. A patient asks her doctor how long she has left to live. The brutally honest doctor replies, "Three months." A student asks his friend what he thinks of his art project. The friend replies, "The horse looks too big." In both examples, the answer comes as a shock. Yes, the person asked. Yes, you answered the question. But the answer comes blasting out like a bullet, and there is little time for the person listening to be prepared.

In gentle honesty, you give the person the answer, but you also give the person time to be prepared to hear it. You can do this in two ways that can be used together or separately.

1. Start by saying some positive things and then talk about the difficult news.
2. Discuss facts that lead the person to the bad news. Take him through the story of what happened, right up to the point of the bad news. In this approach you want him to start guessing in his mind the sad ending, even before you say it.

Look at the examples below. The gentle part of the answer is in italics and put inside the parenthesis.

What do you think of my art project?
(Hey, this is really different. I love the way you've done the shading and the colors for the trees. The only thing I'm wondering about, is that maybe) the horse looks too big.

How long do I have to live?
(Well, as you know, we decided to stop the chemotherapy. I think this was a good decision for you, as you can spend time with your family without the chemotherapy making you feel sicker. Like last weekend when you were with your grandchildren. I know they'll treasure this time. You did everything you could to stop the cancer, with the surgery and chemotherapy. But it only works for 1/3 of patients with your type of cancer. Now that we've stopped treatment, we are probably looking at around) three months.

ANSWERS THAT WILL HURT THE PERSON, AND ARE NOT IMPORTANT FOR THE PERSON TO KNOW, SHOULD BE GIVEN TO MEET THE PERSON'S CURRENT NEED

I don't understand why people get so angry when I answer their questions.

When you know that an answer will hurt a person, it is important to ask yourself, "What does the person need from me right now?" If you are a doctor, and your patient is asking you how long she has to live, she needs an answer so she can make plans and prepare. If your friend is in the middle of an art project, and he is looking for your artistic advice on how to improve it, he needs to know which parts to change.

But if your grandmother is dying, and she has explicitly told her family that she would like to spend her last few days with a sense of normalcy, as though she will be around for another 10 years, then when you ask yourself, "What does she need right now?" Your answer should be something like, "to pretend that everything is normal." This may not be how you would choose to cope with dying, and it may feel very wrong to you, but it's her death and she has the right to do it her way.

When she says, "Let's make plans for Christmas."

You can reply, "Sure Grandma, what would you like to do?" rather than, "You won't be with us for Christmas."

When you answer to meet your grandmother's needs you are not lying or saying she will be here. You are just showing her that you can give her what she needs, to spend her last few months helping her feel that everything is normal and okay.

The following examples explore the question, "What does the person need from me right now?"

You're at an art night looking at your child's or friend's art which is up on the wall. He's drawn a picture of trees, hills, and a horse. The horse looks too big.

	NEEDS	ANSWER	HOW THE ARTIST FEELS
YOU FORGET ABOUT WHAT THE PERSON NEEDS AND JUST ANSWER THE QUESTION	He needs praise and to feel encouraged.	You give a truthful answer that does not meet the need. "Well the horse is way too big."	He feels sad and defeated. He looks around the room and notices how everyone else has a friend or parent who is saying nice things about their art. He decides that his art must be really bad. He feels less confident next time to try something new.
YOU ASK YOURSELF, "WHAT DOES THE PERSON NEED FROM ME RIGHT NOW?"	He needs praise and to feel encouraged.	You give a truthful answer that meets the need. "I love the colors, and your trees look so realistic."	He feels encouraged and cared for. He might decide that art isn't really his thing, but he feels the confidence to try again, or to try something else.

Consciously Learn The Unwritten Rules

Your friend is about to give a big presentation. Just before she goes on stage she turns to you and asks, "How do I look?" You know that she's worked hard on the presentation, but her suit looks wrinkled.

	NEEDS	ANSWER	HOW YOUR FRIEND FEELS
YOU FORGET ABOUT WHAT THE PERSON NEEDS AND JUST ANSWER THE QUESTION	She needs to increase her confidence, and to reduce anxiety.	You give a truthful answer that does not meet the need. "Did you iron your suit? It looks wrinkled."	Her anxiety goes even higher, and her confidence lower. She messes up the first part of her presentation. Later, when thinking about things, she decides that you might have made her feel bad on purpose. She wonders if you're after her job and decides not to trust you anymore.
YOU ASK YOURSELF, "WHAT DOES THE PERSON NEED FROM ME RIGHT NOW?"	She needs to increase her confidence, and to reduce anxiety.	You give a truthful answer that meets the need. "You look like you're about to give an amazing presentation."	Your friend feels more confident, and less anxious. She feels fortunate to have you on the team.

CARING FOR OTHERS

PRACTICE COGNITIVE CARING

My clients often share that they care about others, but they have difficulties feeling other people's emotions. One client, Anna, described how she found it challenging to support her brother while he was going through a divorce. She understood why her brother was sad and felt bad about his situation, but she didn't feel sad. What she normally felt was anxious. Anna worried that her facial expressions looked too happy, or that family members would discover that she wasn't actually feeling his pain. At times, she would try to pull up a sad memory of her own so that she could cry when he was crying.

Other clients note how they struggle to feel people's happiness and are criticized for having facial expressions that look too neutral. Some people feel other people's feelings deeply. Others don't. For those who don't:

- Know that you're not alone. There are many others who care about people in a cognitive rather than a feeling way.
- Take the time to explain your perspective to family or friends who you can trust. For example, "I'm so sorry about the loss of your job. It's hard for me to feel other people's emotions, but I know it's a difficult time for you."
- Communicate that you want to help and support the person. "I'm here to help in any way I can."
- Ways to cognitively care include anything you can think of – handing someone a tissue or a glass of water, cooking a meal, driving someone, organizing something for them, sharing an idea to solve the problem, using words to communicate that you understand their challenge.
- Be aware of the possible strengths of cognitive caring, such as working in a hospital emergency room where action is required despite all the strong emotions.

ARRIVE AT A PARTY 10 MINUTES AFTER THE GIVEN TIME

Your supervisor might like it when you show up early for work, but arriving early for a party can be considered rude and cause stress for the host. It can also put you in the uncomfortable position of having to make conversation with the host all by yourself. Arriving 10 minutes after the given time will help your host to be ready, and help will you to not be alone.

JUST BECAUSE HOSTS ARE BEING NICE TO YOU DOES NOT MEAN THAT THEY WANT YOU TO STAY

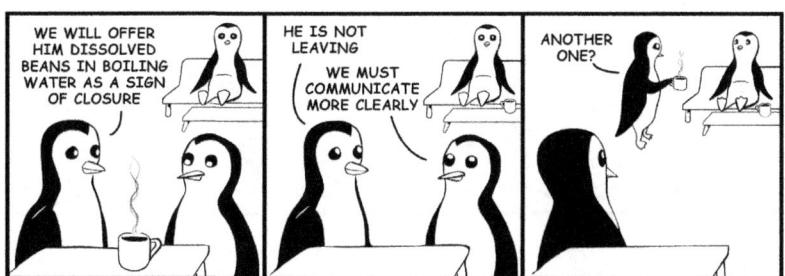

People on the spectrum are often very good at arriving at an event on time, but are less successful at knowing when to leave. A friend or host might continue to talk to you, give you something to drink, smile, and listen to what you have to say, all while thinking to themselves, "I really want them to leave!"

While this may seem rather confusing, you must remember that they view it as their job to keep you happy while you are in their home. Your job is to know when to leave.

IT'S TIME TO LEAVE A PARTY OR EVENT WHEN AROUND 50% OF THE GUESTS HAVE LEFT

When you keep this rule, you will not be leaving an event early or late but will be leaving at the same time as the average guest. In this case, average is good.

NEVER TELL A CHILD THAT SANTA, THE EASTER BUNNY, OR THE TOOTH FAIRY AREN'T REAL. ALWAYS DISCUSS IT WITH YOUR PARTNER BEFORE TELLING YOUR OWN CHILD

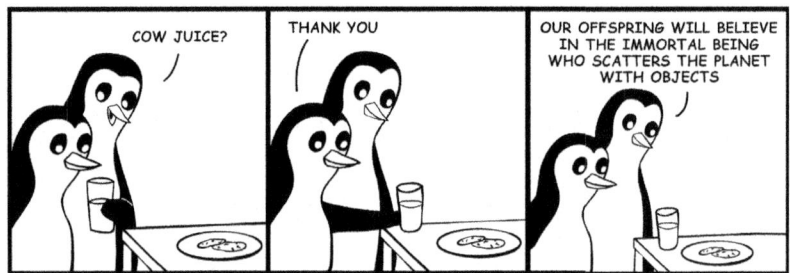

Children are very good at knowing who will tell them the truth, and no matter what age you are they might think that you will give them an honest answer to their "Is Santa real?" question. But you need to remember that it's not your secret to tell. This is the job of their parents.

If you are a parent, then always discuss it with your partner first. If you don't, you will probably receive an angry response like, "You did what?" This is not because your partner doesn't want you to be honest, but because telling the truth about these mythical beings represents an end to childhood innocence.

Ways to answer the question while still being honest include phrases such as, "That's an interesting question!" "Well, I hear Santa lives at the North Pole, and I've never been there." "I think I saw a bunny hopping around outside once."

WHEN YOU BUY A PRESENT, BE SURE YOU ARE BUYING SOMETHING THE OTHER PERSON WILL WANT, RATHER THAN SOMETHING YOU WANT

For many autistic people gift giving can be incredibly stressful. I have clients who have been told they are not a good friend because they chose the wrong item or they failed to give a gift because they didn't know what to buy. When purchasing a gift, don't assume that your spouse or work colleague will be as thrilled as you to own something that you are interested in. Look for signs that the person may want something including:

- They linger over an object in a store or online and express a liking for it.
- They express a liking for something that someone else has.
- They mention a need. "This would be so much faster if I had a ..."
- For romantic gifts, avoid items that are considered a part of household chores, such as a vacuum cleaner or a dishwasher.
- A gift card can be an excellent choice, especially for someone you don't know well.
- If you're not sure what someone wants, ask.

DO ONE KIND ACT FOR A FAMILY MEMBER EACH DAY

Neurotypicals like to see that their family members love them. If they don't see evidence of your love on a regular basis, you are likely to hear statements such as, "I know that you love me, but you just never show it," "You seem to be so self-involved," or "You only care about yourself."

Hearing these statements can be confusing and lead to withdrawal or feeling as if you "will never be good at that sort of thing." Fortunately, the solution is very simple: follow the rule above and do one kind act for a family member every day. Make a conscious choice to include it as part of your daily routine, and your family life and relationships will greatly improve. Just be sure to vary what you do and who you are doing it for, so that nobody in your household feels left out.

The acts do not need to be time-consuming; small things go a long way. For example, several children have told me how a hug, kind word, or gesture of support from their parent with autism means so much to them, especially if they have had difficulty connecting with this parent. Think about the different things you can do:

- Send an encouraging text. ("I hope your ... goes well.")
- Cook a favorite meal.
- Prepare a soda/ coffee/ tea.
- Write a short note and leave it somewhere to be found later on. Elementary school children love finding notes from their parents in their lunch boxes ("Have a great lunch").
- Hide a small inexpensive gift in a bag or suitcase with a note saying that it's from you.
- Offer to help with something. It doesn't matter if the person says no; it's the offering that makes an impact.

BOUNDARIES

IT'S OKAY TO SAY NO

When someone asks you if you want to do something, you have the choice between two answers: yes and no. It's okay to say no.

Many people on the spectrum feel compelled to say yes if they think that's what the other person wants. For some, this comes from years of being taught to "be nice to people." For others, it arises out of a fear of coping with the social consequences of disappointing someone. People can become sad, pushy, or angry when told no, and for a person on the spectrum, it can be easier to just say yes than to be on the receiving end of these emotions.

It's important to remember that when someone asks you a yes/no question, it's usually because the person doesn't know the answer. Would you like to go to the movies tonight? Do you like Indian food? Should we go to the pool? Do you want to get married?

You don't need to try and guess what answer they are looking for. Just tell them what you are thinking. If you are thinking no, then the correct answer is no. To become more comfortable with saying no:

- Start to practice saying "No" in less stressful situations where you might not see the person again. For example, say "No" at the store register when asked if you want to give your email, phone number, or get the special credit card.
- Tell the person you would like some time to think it over. This will allow you to come out of what might feel like a pressured situation and give your answer when you feel ready.
- Avoid indirect answers such as "Maybe later," "Next time," or "I'd love to but I can't because..." This will only make the person ask you again.
- Keep your tone of voice kind, calm, and firm.
- Remember that in healthy relationships you are allowed to say "No."

IF YOU'RE NOT IN LAW ENFORCEMENT, DON'T POLICE OTHERS

*I like to follow the rules and punish
anyone who doesn't keep them.*

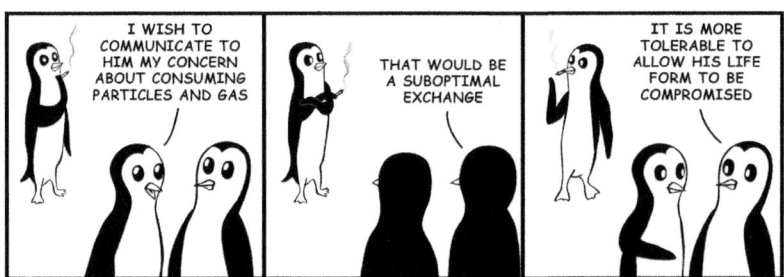

When you like rules it can be very difficult to watch other people breaking them. It can make you feel anxious, angry, or personally responsible for correcting the situation. This can be especially true at school, work, or in a setting where there is something that you are passionate about. Seeing other people "doing it wrong" can tempt you to step in and tell others just how it's supposed to be done.

For children, policing others often involves correcting peers who are breaking rules such as not taking off their shoes, or correcting those who are talking in class when the teacher has asked for silence. Policing can also be directed at adults who are doing things such as smoking or eating unhealthy foods. Many parents tell me how their children have approached a stranger on the street with, "You shouldn't smoke; it will kill you."

While wanting things done the right way is a good characteristic, policing others is not. Take care of your own behavior and let other people take care of theirs. And remember, in policing others when you shouldn't, you too are breaking a rule and "doing it wrong."

FAITH DOES NOT HAVE TO BE BASED ON FEELINGS

*Enthusiasm is hard to fake as it's a different kind of smile.
I don't always feel it.*

It can be difficult when faith is an important part of your life but you struggle to feel God's presence. You might have little emotional connection to religious services, prayer, meditation, or religious texts. When others around you are leaking their emotions in your place of worship and expecting you to do the same, I want you to set a healthy boundary and remember that your faith can be done your way, and does not have to be based on feelings.

Many of my clients with a strong cognitive faith have found meaning in memorizing text, teaching, volunteering, thought-filled prayer, caring for others, religious music, and art. If anyone has a problem with the way your mind is made, simply remind the person that you are the created, not the creator.

PEOPLE WILL RESPECT YOU MORE IF THEY CAN'T TAKE ADVANTAGE OF YOU

People on the spectrum are often taken advantage of. This includes being bullied, having things stolen, being asked to work extra hours, not getting credit for work, being pressured into helping people who are mean, not being paid, and being forced to buy things under pressure.

While wanting other people to like you can make it hard to set limits, the truth is that people will respect you more when they can't take advantage of you. If someone is only interested in using you, then it's better that he or she is not in your life. To protect yourself:

- Never lend a person more money than you are willing to give, as it might not be returned.

- Beware of mean people who suddenly become nice.
- Before starting a new job or hiring someone for a project, always clarify the contract.
- Know that your time is valuable too.
- When possible, put things in written form, such as an email.
- Give yourself at least 24 hours to think about difficult decisions. ("Let me think about that, and I'll get back to you.")
- Involve people in authority (tell the teacher someone took your lunch, ask the manager if you should keep working on your project or do the one your co-worker dropped on your desk).
- Ask a trusted friend or family member for advice.

USE SOCIAL STORIES FOR CHILDREN

When I'm writing or reading I can picture it like a movie. I can zoom in on a detail and zoom out.

I have included this rule for people who are working with children on the spectrum because it's a powerful and effective way to teach rules and help children understand boundaries. Even after years of experience, I'm still surprised at how children enjoy the process of writing a social story, and how quickly their behavior can change when this technique is used.

Social stories teach behaviors by telling a story about the importance of following a specific rule. They have context, details, and include the child's own unique experiences. Children can picture themselves in the situation and will run through the scenario in their minds. It is interesting, colorful, and has texture.

To better understand the impact of telling a story, imagine that I told you, "When you are driving and come to a light that is turning red, you must slow down and stop." My telling you this will probably have no effect on your behavior the next time you come to a light. You might not even remember that I had said it.

Now imagine that I said, "I was driving my car and when I came to a light that was turning red, I decided to speed up and run through it. I had a friend in my car sitting next to me, and all of a sudden this van drove right towards me and went into the passenger's door. I don't think I'll ever forget the horrid crashing sound, and I looked over and saw that my friend was trapped.

We were both crying, and the ambulance had to take her to the hospital. She had a broken leg and a broken arm. You know, the rule is when you come to a light that is turning red, slow down and stop. If you keep the rule, everyone in the car will be safe and happy."

My telling you this story, especially if it were true, will probably encourage you to slow down the next time you come to a yellow light.

There is no one way to write a social story, but the stories I write all use the same format:

- The child is involved as much as possible in the process. Even children who do not appear to be interested can make small choices about how it is written. By participating in the story's creation they will be much more likely to accept the rule.

    "Let's write a story about this.
    Which way should we put the paper?
    What should the story be called?
    What color marker do you want to use for the title?
    What happens first? Then what happens?
    Can you draw a picture of what happens?
    I've drawn a picture. Can you help me color it?
    I'm so glad you're helping, I'm terrible at art."

- There is always a title. As this will be used when you want to refer to the rule it is helpful to have it describe the specific situation. Keep the title short enough that you can quickly mention it if a challenging situation arises. "Do you remember the . . . story? Now, what was that rule?"

>Examples of titles include:
>When my Class Gets Noisy.
>Brushing my teeth.
>Playing with my friend.

- The first paragraph describes the behavior that is happening now.
  >Start with what causes the behavior and include the location if it usually happens in one particular place. I like to use the words "Sometimes" or "I might," so that the child knows it does not always happen this way. (Sometimes I'm at school, and the class gets very noisy.) Then describe what he does and why this is a bad choice. (I might start screaming and run out of the room. This makes my friends angry as they don't like my screaming. My teacher isn't happy as she has to stop teaching and come get me.)

- The second paragraph defines the new rule.
  >THE RULE IS . . . This should be written in capital letters, and with a bright color like red. Clearly write the rule. Be sure that it is concrete, specific, and that it states what to do.
  >If a child is only told what he shouldn't be doing, he will get stuck when the situation occurs. "Don't scream," doesn't tell him what to do. "I must behave," tells him what to do but is too abstract, as "behave" can mean many different things. "Ask an adult for help," gives clear directions.

- The last paragraph is the happy ending.
  >This is the ending that happens when the rule is kept. I usually include a statement about how proud the parents or teachers will be and how he will feel.

Consciously Learn The Unwritten Rules

Once the social story is written, there are several things you can do to help reinforce the rule and practice the new behavior:

- Read the story together.

    Ask questions while trying to keep it fun. What's the rule again? Is it to go screaming out of the room?

- Act out the story.

    You can switch roles so that sometimes you're the child. Tell him you're going to do it the wrong way, and see if he can catch your mistake. Film him doing it right and have him play it back. Each time he watches himself, it reinforces what he can do.

- Print several copies of the story.

    Keep a copy in a folder at home with other social stories, and keep a copy in the environments where the behavior occurs. You can also take a photo of the story with your phone, so you can pull it up at any time.

- Read the story to the child before entering the situation that causes the behavior.

    You want to focus most of your teaching before the situation occurs so that he has a greater chance of being successful. If your child forgets what to do, point to the story and say, "Now what's that rule again? What are we supposed to do?" Look at the paper with your child, as if you are also trying to remember.

- Establish that it is the rule that is telling him what to do, not you.

    "I don't want to ask my teacher!"
    "Well the rule says . . ."

On the following pages are two examples of social stories illustrated by children.

AUTISM RULES

WHEN MY CLASS GETS NOISY

Sometimes I'm at school, and the class gets very noisy. I might start screaming and run out of the room. This makes my friends angry as they don't like my screaming. My teacher isn't happy as she has to stop teaching and come get me.

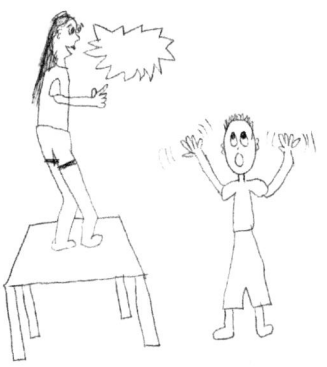

THE RULE IS: WHEN THE CLASS IS TOO NOISY I WILL ASK MY TEACHER IF I CAN PUT ON MY HEADPHONES.

When I keep the rule and put on my headphones, my ears won't hurt from all the noise. My teacher and friends will be happy. My mom and dad will be proud of me, and I will be happy too.

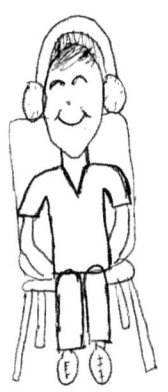

Consciously Learn The Unwritten Rules

POLICING OTHERS

People in my class sometimes break the rules. They might talk when the teacher said to be quiet, or they wear their shoes on the mat. I might tell them, "Stop talking," or "You can't wear shoes. Take them off." When I tell people what to do, they get angry with me. My teacher is also angry at me.

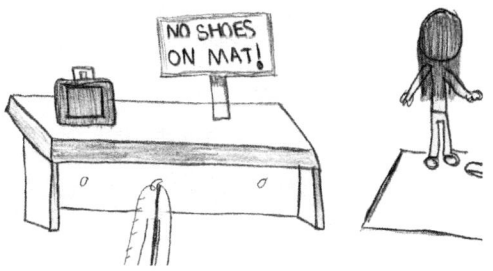

THE RULE IS: WHEN I SEE PEOPLE BREAKING THE RULES, I WILL REMEMBER THAT IT'S NOT MY JOB TO CORRECT THEM. I WILL IGNORE IT AND GET BACK TO WHAT I'M DOING.

When I keep the rule, my friends and teacher will be happy with me. My mom and dad will be proud of me, and I will be happy too.

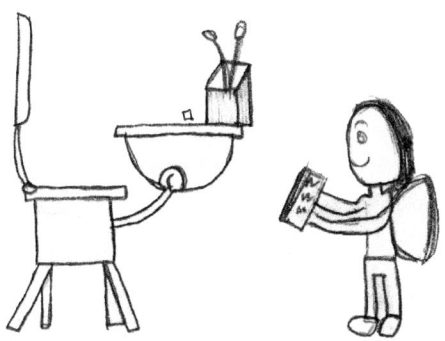

AUTISM RULES

CHAPTER 3

Strengthen Your Social Radar

I'm bad at parking my car. And I mean really bad. One time in Hawaii, I was lucky enough to be just behind a car that had pulled out of a parking spot next to the beach on a late Friday afternoon. This is a time when many people go swimming, and I had expected to wait for twenty minutes or more. It was a parallel parking spot on a narrow curved road. I signaled that I was going to park and the traffic behind me stopped. The traffic in front of me stopped, and a family walking next to me waved for me to go ahead. They would wait to cross the street.

I took a deep breath. Thoughts of, "I can do this" battled with "No I can't, and everyone's watching." I tried to remember what my father had taught me, something about lining my car up with the car in front and making a sharp turn with the wheel. I made a first attempt and failed. The end of the car was in, but the front half was sticking out. I pulled back out and tried again, failing with similar results. I made a third attempt and failed again. I kept trying. I kept failing. Everyone was staring. I felt my heart racing and my hands getting sweaty. But I kept trying and failing. Eventually, after about five minutes that felt like an hour, a young man tapped on my window and asked if he could park my car for me. Humiliated and thankful, I accepted, jumping out of the car as fast as I could. In one swift move, he maneuvered my car into the space, turned off the engine, and handed me the keys.

Everyone has weaknesses.

In this chapter, you will learn how you can strengthen your social radar, so that no matter what the situation, you will have the skills to succeed without someone having to leap into your world and do it for you.

IT'S HARD FOR YOU TO KNOW WHAT YOUR RADAR IS NOT PICKING UP

I'm astounded by how easy socializing is for some people.

Each time I attempted to park my car, I hoped that I could correct my errors from my previous failures. But it wasn't until I finished maneuvering that I realized I had gone wrong again. I was not where I was supposed to be, and the other drivers looked frustrated. Many of my clients describe similar experiences in social situations. They keep going with a conversation or a behavior, hoping that it will turn out well, only to find that after all their efforts, they have made an error and someone is angry with them.

One of the most important first steps in strengthening your social radar is to accept that you may lack the perspective to catch your own mistakes. I could only see the world around me from my position inside the car; I didn't have the skills to know how turning the wheel a certain way would affect the outcome, and I wasn't thinking clearly because I was anxious.

It's the same for many autistic people in social situations. They can't see themselves as other people see them, they may lack the skills to fully understand how their actions will affect the outcome, and their thinking can be compromised due to anxiety.

You will make significantly more progress in strengthening your social radar when you can find a way to look at yourself through the eyes of another person.

CHOOSE A SOCIAL GUIDE FOR YOUR RADAR

*I feel like I was meant to be a woodland creature,
but I'm here with the humans.*

Everyone has guides. Luke Skywalker had Yoda. The Karate Kid had Mr. Miyagi. You might have parents, teachers, managers, pastors, tour guides, fitness coaches, GPS systems, or apps. Guides are everywhere.

When you are on the spectrum, you will need a social guide. This is someone who will help you see yourself as others see you. A social guide can be a family member, friend, teacher, peer, counselor, or manager. The person should be someone you trust, who can be objective, and who has good social skills. You can have several social guides, each specializing in a different kind of situation. For example, you might have a friend at work, an uncle at family gatherings, and a counselor who you can visit for advice.

A social guide can:

- Help you make sense of situations that did not turn out the way you expected.
- Advise you on how to approach upcoming events.
- Explain the strange behavior of the neurotypical.
- Let you know if you are being taken advantage of.
- Help you set goals to develop your skills.
- Give you feedback on how you did in a social situation. Feedback should be concrete, not abstract. "You were rude," is abstract. It doesn't tell you where you went wrong. "Wait until everyone is sitting down before you start to eat," is concrete. It tells you exactly where you made your mistake.

It's important to remember that this is your guide. You get to decide who you want to help you and why. For parents who might be choosing guides for their child, be sure to involve them in the decisions when possible. Does your child have a favorite teacher? Is there a special instructor of an activity your child would like to be better at?

A social guide can be a wonderful resource for strengthening your social radar, but they come with a couple of warnings. The first warning concerns dependence. The guide's primary role is to help you be independently successful at social situations. You should notice that you are getting better at thinking through social situations on your own, that you are having more successful outcomes even when your guide is not around, and that you are taking on new social roles and attending new events. What you don't want to see is that you are calling up your guide every time you have a problem. If a guide is working with your child, try to avoid your child looking to their guide when asked a question.

The second warning concerns boundaries. It's essential that you communicate to your guide how and when you would like to be helped.

You don't want to feel overwhelmed by their feedback. But you also don't want a guide who doesn't step up to help you when you need it. To solve the boundary issue, set clear expectations around what type of help you would like. Remember that you can't improve all of your social skills at once. Have a look at these examples of clear expectations:

- A half-hour meeting once a month to discuss one thing I did better at and one thing I need to work on.
- Let me know if I've upset someone in the office or classroom, and what I can do about it. Don't tell me about more than one person or situation a week.
- Just text me if I'm doing something weird.
- Can we meet once a month so I can ask you questions about how neurotypicals think?
- Can you give me feedback after the group project meeting on how I did with my non-verbal communication, specifically eye-contact and tone of voice?
- I'm going to be organizing the social event. Could we meet two weeks before it so that I can get your help on what I need to do?

SOCIAL RADARS ARE MAINLY VISUAL

It feels wrong to make eye contact, so I take off my glasses and then I don't feel the judgment from blurry people.

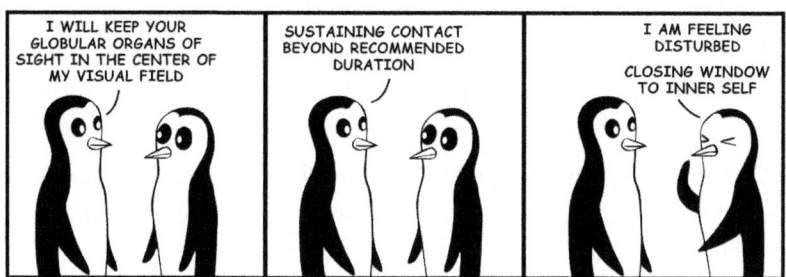

Most information transmitted to the brain is visual, and neurons for visual activity take up more gray matter than touch and hearing combined. In other words, many of our decisions, judgments, and feelings are based more on what we see in the world rather than what we hear, smell, or touch.

One young man I worked with was excellent at expressing his thoughts and feelings. However, whenever he talked, he either held his eye contact for too long or he looked down at the floor. For his peers, this was a deal-breaker. It didn't matter how thoughtful or intelligent he was, his eye contact made others feel uncomfortable. Even though this may seem unjust, it is a reality. If what you are doing looks too different from others, you are at greater risk of being judged negatively.

The good news is that many people on the spectrum are excellent at visual processing. They can often replay scenes from a movie in their mind or recall details from a photograph. This gift can be used to strengthen your social radar.

When you walk into a social event, a lot of information will be coming at you from other senses, more than the typical person (flashing lights, humming sounds from the air conditioning, itchy clothes, strong smells). Because of this information overload, you will need to make a conscious effort to focus on the visual information. Study what the people look like they are doing. Analyze it like you would a series of numbers, notes of music, or lines of computer coding.

Although you may be tempted to start with the smaller details of what you are seeing (one of the chairs is a different style), be sure to start by taking a larger look at the whole scene (employees at the office lunch meeting). Then break it down into parts (the women are in one area). Then study the smaller details (people only have drinks, nobody has started the buffet). Following the steps in order will help to ensure that you do not get caught up in the details, only to miss the big picture.

Once you have a visual understanding of the scene, you can choose what you would like to do. Keep your actions similar to those of other people (go stand in the line for a soda, don't pick up a plate for the buffet).

Neurotypicals unconsciously do this when they walk into a social event. You will be thinking about it before you go somewhere and when you are there. But after a while it will become more natural, and like learning to read, you'll find yourself doing it without much effort.

The following two charts show what type of information is included in each of the steps. The first chart is for helping a child. You may want to take the chart with you when you go somewhere or take a picture of it with your phone so you have it when needed. Ask the child if he can "win the game by finding all four steps." Read the first step, and ask questions that will help lead him in his processing. Be sure to encourage his developing skills, "You're so good at this." You can also reward him with a prize when he wins the game.

The second chart is for adults. To strengthen your social radar, you will want to memorize the chart to remind yourself to process the information. Take note of which steps are harder for you, which ones you find more interesting, and which you are more likely to forget.

ORDER OF PROCESSING FOR CHILDREN	EXAMPLES OF QUESTIONS TO HELP CHILDREN PROCESS
1. BIG PICTURE	What's the big picture? Whose birthday is it? Why are we meeting today? Why is it called a Thanksgiving meal? What are we celebrating today?
2. PARTS	Can you see the two different groups? Do you see your friends? Did you notice the kids aren't in this room? It's only parents. Look at that group over there. What are they doing?
3. DETAILS	Can you tell me some details? What are those kids holding in their hands? Are your friends inside also playing with water balloons? Everyone's looking at the same picture in the book. What page is it?
4. CHOOSE WHAT I WANT TO DO	What would you like to do? Who would you like to play with? Where do you want to sit? What looks interesting to you? Remember what you noticed about how they are playing (no water balloons inside).

AUTISM RULES

ORDER OF PROCESSING FOR ADULTS	DESCRIPTION OF STEPS FOR ADULTS
1. BIG PICTURE	This is a general understanding of what you are seeing. It's essential to grasp the big picture in order to adjust to the event. What type of event is it? Is it public, private, a planned meeting? What is the location? Who is present? What is the purpose of the event?
2. PARTS	Divide the larger scene into parts, noting common factors that bring different groups together. Common factors might include specific roles people have, age, gender, interest in certain activities, familiarity with others.
3. DETAILS	Bring your focus to the smaller details. This is where you will often find the unwritten social rules. What are the hands doing? Where are people looking? Did people take off their coats? Where did they put them? Are people close together or spread out?
4. CHOOSE WHAT I WANT TO DO	Choose a group or individual you would like to join. Walk over and join a group. Be aware of the details you have noticed (you don't arrive with a plate of food if people only have drinks).

LEARN FROM THOSE WHO HAVE GONE BEFORE YOU

I know some people can just read about something and then do it, but I need to watch others doing it first.

When I was younger I once questioned my artistic sister about why she was spending hours copying drawings, rather than designing her own. I can't remember her reply, but it probably involved going behind the sofa where she usually went to draw in peace. That same sister is now a very successful artist who has worked on movies including Kung Fu Panda and Peter Pan. A fact she knew at a very young age, which I had failed to grasp, is that learning from others is an important part of developing any skill.

In addition to strengthening the visual information when you are in social situations, it's also helpful for you to study and copy social skills outside the demands of a social situation. When you're not in the social situation your anxiety will be lower, and you'll be better able to process what you're seeing without having to worry about how you're doing.

There are several ways of developing these skills by learning from others who have gone before you:

- Look for pictures and videos online for previous years of the same event and similar events.
- If possible, attend an event or similar event as an observer before you participate.
- To help you process the information, imagine yourself in the scene.
- Try to predict what's going to happen next and notice the details that reveal the unwritten social rules.
- Study body language, facial expressions, and tone of voice.

TURN THE BACKGROUND VOLUME DOWN

*When there's a bunch of sound,
it feels like a knife stabbing.*

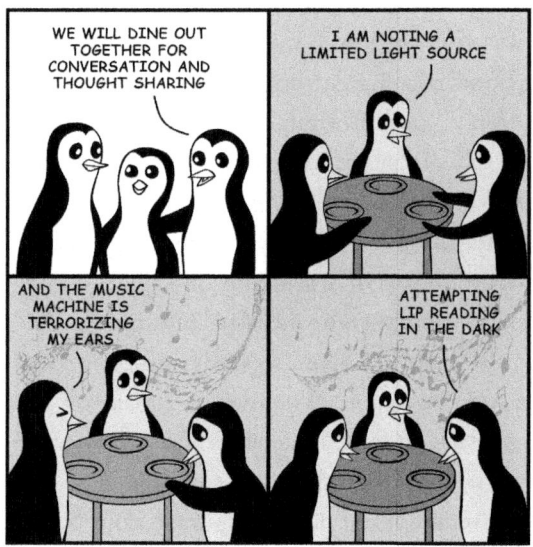

Imagine for a moment that you are listening to a friend who has an accent that is difficult to understand. While she speaks, there is a group of people standing next to you, talking to you at the same time. Some of the people in the group speak louder and clearer than your friend.

As you try to listen to your friend, your mind uses a lot of energy to sort through the information from the loud, clear people, even though you're not interested in what they are saying. Your mind processes the group's conversation and remembers it. Through all of their noise and information, you try to grasp what your friend is saying.

For many of you on the spectrum, learning new social skills is very similar to this situation. Like listening to a person with an unfamiliar accent, it can require concentration and focus, but there can be a lot of background noise, making it hard to process the important information.

The background noise is all of the information coming from your sensory system. You might have been taught that we only have the five senses of sight, sound, taste, touch and smell, but we actually have more including balance (vestibular) and body awareness (proprioception). For the neurotypical person, this sensory information enters the mind without too much distraction. For example, a neurotypical person mind might hear the hum of an air conditioner, decide that it's not important information, and then block it out to focus on someone speaking.

When you are autistic, this blocking out doesn't happen as easily. The sensory information remains chatting, and often shouting in the background. You might smell something horrible and all you can do is think about it and wonder why it isn't bothering anyone else (the answer is that they haven't even noticed it). You might be focused on the sight of a crooked painting, badly placed tile, or lighting that is too dark (other people haven't noticed these either).

It is also possible that you hear conversations in the background too clearly, distracting you from what the person beside you is saying, or you feel an itch from your clothes or pain from a gentle touch on the arm.

Even the taste of food can become an unwanted distraction if its texture is not what you expect. Some of my clients have a hard time standing still and an equally hard time avoiding bumping into people due to challenges with body awareness. It's not surprising that it can be difficult to pay attention to your social radar with all this sensory background noise.

One person who describes these challenges is Dawn Prince-Hughes, an accomplished anthropologist whose photographic memory allows her to remember her past with remarkable clarity (Prince-Hughes, 2005). She didn't realize that she had autism until the age of thirty-six, so many of the things she experienced growing up were confusing to her, especially the way she processed her sensory information.

For Dawn, sights, sounds, and touch felt more like a jumbled, knotted mess that needed to be avoided, rather than information that could teach her about the world and make her feel safe. As a toddler, the floor didn't ground her but made her so uncomfortable that she tried to avoid crawling by clinging onto furniture. When people cuddled her, it wasn't a safe cocoon for absorbing love, but a space that gave her the sensation of drowning. Even dust between her toes sent her into a tantrum.

School was especially difficult for her. In noisy classrooms, the sounds pounded against her ears and the lights felt like piercing blinding whiteness. Numbers also had specific colors. If she added seven, which she processed as being green, and three, which was blue, she would get blue-green, which happened to be nine.

Dawn explains, "On a sensory level, public school is a real nightmare. It smells bad, the clanking of the lockers are loud, the halls make noise reverberate. You sit in a hard chair at a hard desk looking at a hard chalkboard" (Prince-Hughes, 2015).

It is often difficult for those of us who are not on the spectrum to understand how overwhelming the sensory noise can be. We might see a child sitting at her desk not doing her work, or an adult standing alone at a party and have no idea of their sensory chaos. This is exactly what happened to Dawn. Her third-grade teacher thought she was arrogant, lazy, and loud. She believed her parents had spoiled her, and she assigned extra work, used a stopwatch for tests, and screamed loudly. This had the effect of terrifying Dawn and made her feel as if she was in a sensory whirlwind.

To turn the background noise down, it's important that you first become aware of what your sensory challenges are. Review the sensorimotor list in Chapter 4, and note which areas are relevant for you. Under each area, you will see examples of how to cope by making changes to the environment or to yourself. For example, if you have a sensitivity to bright lights, you can change to halogen lighting or wear sunglasses. You can also inform other people of your sensory issues. The more others understand your needs, the better they will be able to help you. A teacher or manager might be able to put your desk in a quiet area or allow you to wear an adapted version of a uniform. I have also known people who have worked at night to avoid the sensory overload of a bustling office.

Dawn Prince-Hughes eventually found a unique way to turn her sensory noise down while strengthening her social radar. She started to go to her local zoo and sit on a bench in front of a glass window to watch a group of gorillas. The glass barrier between herself and the animals allowed her to be on the outside of the experience in a place that had no expectations for interactions and was away from the sensory chaos. She didn't have to listen to others talking to her or worry about missing an important cue. She didn't have to be stressed about responding or cope with being touched. She could simply observe.

Being with the animals from a distance reminded her of some of the better memories of her childhood, like lying in bed and hearing the sounds of her family in the morning or seeing her family through the window from the outside of her house. During these times she had felt happy, safe, and even closer to her family than if she had been in the same room. These feelings came back to her in the secure and calm enclosure of the zoo, and she sat silently for hours recording and studying the gorillas' social interactions. Slowly, she began to see herself in them, and in this quiet space, for the first time in her life, she saw herself in other people too.

DEVELOP A SENSORY DIET

Imagine an eating version of dragging your nails across a chalkboard, but it's in your throat.

Feeling balanced is important for both our physical and mental health. For example, when you feel hungry you eat, and when you're tired you sleep. In the same way, when there is too much sensory noise, your system will become unbalanced. Sensory input from sounds, smells, light, taste, touch, and unpredictable people can cause a feeling of chaos, and it will become natural to seek out activities to help you recover. These activities are like reaching for a glass of iced water on a hot day.

Neurotypicals try to balance their systems all the time. If you look around a room full of people, you will see that they are constantly in movement. They will be shifting, scratching, stretching, chewing gum, nibbling on a pen, tapping fingers, or shaking a foot. All of this movement is their systems self-regulating.

Following a sensory diet does not mean that you restrict your sensory activities, but rather you will set up a daily or weekly routine of activities to meet your sensory needs. The activities that can help you reach equilibrium will vary, but most tend to have some of the following qualities:

- Quietness
- Repetitiveness
- Predictability
- Stimulation
- Deep physical pressure

If the world feels unpredictable, it can be soothing to draw a certain pattern, eat the same breakfast, wear the same clothes, or go the same way to work every day so that you can see that the houses, streets, and signs are still there. If the world is too big, bright, and noisy, it can be calming to cover yourself in a blanket or crawl into a cupboard. When things feel out of order, looking at symmetrical objects can reassure you that everything is in its place. If being with people is exhausting, then sitting with nature or asking repetitive questions that you already know the answer to can be a reprieve. And when the system is overwhelmed, seeking out a tight hug can calm it all down.

To know what activities are helpful for you, an occupational therapist can analyze your sensory system and develop a specific plan. Your therapist might ask you to keep a log of your daily routine and how you feel at home or work.

You can also develop a sensory diet using the list of your checked sensorimotor items from Chapter 4. Do you have sensory challenges in specific areas such as proprioception or sound? Do any of the listed interventions help you? For example, if you find yourself pacing and sounds are irritating, you can schedule a daily walk while listening to your favorite music.

As part of your sensory diet, you can also schedule breaks away from challenging situations. When a room is full of people standing too close to you, then spending ten minutes in a corner reading a book can help balance your system. This can be especially important for children. Many parents of children with autism get calls from noisy school programs such as after-school care and are told that their child has "behavioral problems." In these situations, it is important to consider that there might be a sensory difficulty.

One of my clients had challenges in an after-school program because she kept hitting other children. We taught her social skills, but the behavior continued and she was about to be thrown out, which was especially difficult for her family as both parents worked. Then we put a plan in place where she was allowed to go in a corner of the room and read a book if she was feeling overwhelmed. It was such a simple intervention that required nothing from the staff, and it turned out to be immediately successful.

Below is an example of a sensory diet that can be used for both children and adults.

MORNING
    Walk outside for 15 minutes or go for a run.
    Take a shower and allow the water to massage your back.
    Wear a soft shirt under your office or school uniform.
    Listen to your favorite music.
    Eat a crunchy cereal or food.

DURING THE DAY AT WORK OR SCHOOL
    Carry a heavy bag to work or school.
    Put earbuds in.
    Exercise for 20 minutes at the gym.
    Swing on the playground from monkey bars.
    Eat a lunch brought from home which contains a favorite strong flavor and a chewy snack.
    Spend 10 minutes in a quiet area of the office or in the school library.

EVENING

    Receive a tight hug from a family member.
    Push a grocery cart.
    Suck on a mint or chew gum.
    Swing on a hammock, rope, or swing.
    Lift weights, swim, run, row, or bike.
    Watch a TV show while being covered with a heavy blanket.
    Walk for 10 minutes.
    Take a bubble bath.
    Listen to music.
    Use a vibrating toothbrush.
    Close blackout curtains.
    Sleep under heavy blankets.

TURN THE ANXIETY DOWN BY LEARNING WHAT *TO* DO

My school is infested with talking people, I get really stressed knowing that I have to go back.

Just like sensory information can affect your social radar, so can anxiety. High anxiety makes it hard for you to process what's happening around you and to try new things.

Some people suffer from generalized anxiety, which means that their anxiety is high across several different settings such as at home, in the community, and at work. Others have phobias or fears of specific things. Common phobias that I've seen for autistic people include birds, flying bugs, balloons, loud noises, elevators, characters in movies, and bad weather. Many of these have an element of unpredictability to them. You never know when a balloon might pop or a wasp will sting.

Another type of anxiety that I often see in my clients is social anxiety, which leads to an avoidance of social situations. This is not surprising given that neurotypicals can be unpredictable. We say things we don't mean ("It's raining cats and dogs" or "I smell a rat"), we lie ("I'm fine"), and our social rules are horribly complex.

One man with autism explained his social anxiety to me using the analogy of clowns. Many people are afraid of clowns because their painted faces make it hard to know what they're thinking or feeling. Are they here to make me laugh or scream? Are they happy, aggressive or angry? What lies behind the mask they wear? Because it's difficult to accurately read the emotions of clowns, it's difficult to judge what they're up to. Are these clowns my friends? How should I interact with them? There is even a word for the fear of clowns—coulrophobia.

What if the world was full of clowns? Family, acquaintances, people at work—all clowns with painted-on faces—unknowable human beings. My client perceived all neurotypical people this way. Unpredictable. Hard to read. Anxiety-provoking.

Unfortunately, when you're experiencing anxiety, you might be told to "just calm down." When I was working with students, I would often hear teachers say these words before sending a child out of their class. One day I saw a young boy with autism outside his classroom jumping up and down on his books, and I realized that he didn't know how to be calm. If he knew how, he wouldn't be in the corridor.

A good teacher wouldn't tell a student with dyslexia to "just learn to read;" she would teach him how to overcome the barriers that made it difficult. When dealing with anxiety, we need to do the same—focus on teaching new skills and strategies.

On the following pages are the rules for a four-step plan to end your anxiety. I know that anxiety is incredibly challenging, and whether you are using the plan for yourself or teaching it to someone else, you will want immediate relief. But please resist the temptation to skip to the end steps without doing the initial work, as the skills build on each other.

WHEN ANXIOUS, STEP 1 IS TO RATE YOUR ANXIETY

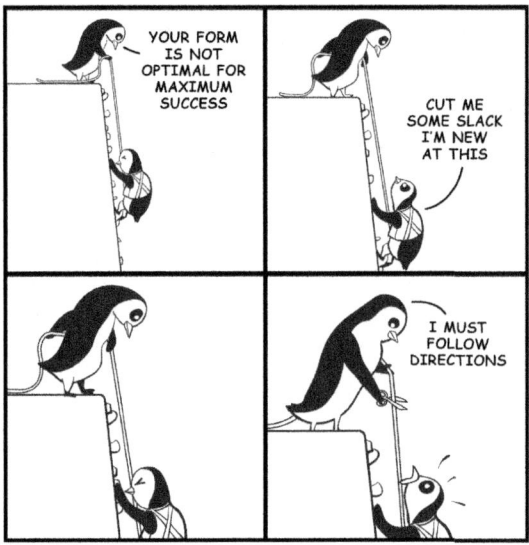

For this first step you will rate your anxiety in different situations. You can do this throughout the day as situations occur or at the end of the day. Keep a note of what happened and what number you were at. Younger children can use a 1-5 scale with pictures next to the numbers. For adults a 1-10 scale works better, with 10 being very anxious and 1 being calm.

Even just mentioning the word "anxiety" can make anxiety increase, but spend a few days on this step. It will help you become aware of the situations that make you the most anxious and help you look for patterns. Is your anxiety worse around certain people or places? Do you first notice it when it gets to a 6 or only when you are already at a 10? When do you feel most relaxed? Remember, it is hard to change something that you're not aware of.

Rating your anxiety will also help you to monitor your progress and communicate your feelings to others. It can be normal for those around you to misjudge how anxious you are, so being able to communicate this quickly and easily by using a number is empowering. In fact, some of my clients find that just being able to label their anxiety with a concrete number starts to give them a sense of control. Take a look at the following rating scale.

10	Very Anxious. Sweaty palms, pounding heart, racing thoughts, arguing, shouting, melting down, withdrawing, leaving.
9	Just on the edge of a meltdown.
8	Anxiety is feeling unmanageable. Hard to think clearly, tense muscles, tight chest, shaking or trembling, shorter and faster breaths from the upper chest.
7	Anxiety has now risen. Thoughts of wanting to leave the situation, worrying about what can go wrong.
6	Anxiety is starting to rise.
5	Neutral.
4	Entering into a comfort zone.
3	Becoming very relaxed. Relaxed muscles, calm, focused, longer and slower breaths.
2	You feel that things are as they should be. No worries about future events, slow heartbeat, calm thoughts.
1	In your calmest state. You might be in a favorite activity or place, content, relaxed, feeling safe.

WHEN ANXIOUS, STEP 2 IS TO UNDERSTAND FIGHT, FLIGHT, FREEZE

I have thousands of worrying things circling in my head that can pop up at any time.

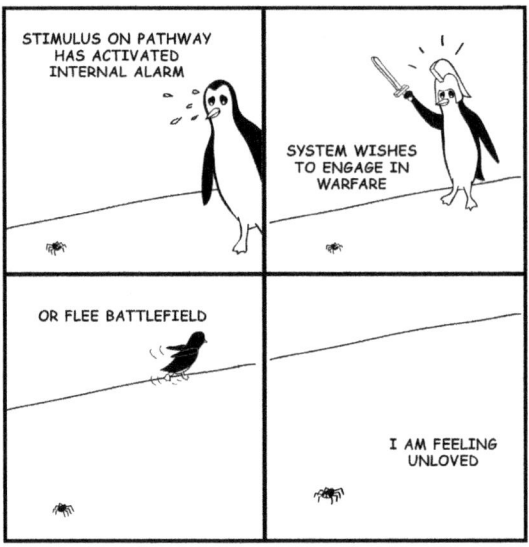

Getting to the higher levels of anxiety can be overwhelming. Common physical responses include sweaty palms, a fast heartbeat, tense muscles, racing thoughts, an upset stomach, shaking, arguing, and wanting to leave. It's like being thrown into the middle of a storm and not knowing what's going on.

Then after the storm passes and the high anxiety subsides, you may find yourself feeling depressed and having thoughts such as, "What's wrong with me?" or "I'll never be okay."

One of the common benefits of having a mind on the autism spectrum is a good memory, especially a visual one. For people with this gift it can also mean replaying a moment of anxiety over and over and obsessing about what went wrong. This usually strengthens the fear and can lead to a phobia for certain situations. Clients will become afraid of the fear itself and say, "I can't go to that shopping mall again," or "I'm afraid I will get anxiety if I go back there." To stop this cycle, it's important to understand what's happening to your body.

For our ancestors who were hunters and gatherers or farmers living off the land in greater isolation, there was an increased chance of being physically attacked. There were wolves, bears, snakes, and threats from both within and between groups of people.

Imagine for a moment that we are living years ago in an isolated area, and we need to get water from a river. On our way to the river a bear approaches and starts to growl at us. We each have a different response. I recognize the danger, but my body feels relaxed, so I stand there for a few seconds wondering what to do. You recognize the danger, but your body sounds an internal alarm that sends out stress hormones. These hormones quickly prepare you to fight the bear, run away (flight), or freeze (hide).

The hormones make your heart beat fast so that blood can be pumped throughout your body for energy. Your muscles become tense for running away or punching the bear. Your mind races to help you make a quick decision—Would it be better to run back to the house, stay to fight, or hide behind a tree? Your stomach aches as your body stops digestion until after the emergency, saving all of its energy for your muscles. You start to sweat as your system tries to keep itself cool in spite of all this activity. Your breathing also changes to shallow upper-chest breaths which increases oxygen. You might also notice that you are shaking. Your chemical alarm is going off. You are in the fight, flight, freeze response.

Your body is shouting at you with everything it's got to fight the bear, or to run away, or to hide. With your quick thinking and extra energy, you run back to the cabin. Now let's pretend that my alarm never did sound. I'm very calm and I don't have much anxiety. I've seen the bear. I'm aware of the danger. I stand there wondering what to do.

Guess who gets eaten for lunch?

When working with children, I will ask them to draw what their bodies look like when they are afraid, and we then label the different parts of their bodies with what is happening and why. For example, "Heart—Beating fast to send oxygen through the body. Feet—Shaky as they want to run away."

The fight or flight response is a mechanism that has helped us to survive for generations. The problem is that the things that set off our alarm nowadays are not usually things we can punch, run away from, or cease to engage in. An employee can't punch his boss when he's given a stressful project or a surprise birthday party. A student can't run out of school as soon as the teacher says that her test is timed. If you could actually run away or hit someone, your body would feel as if it had done its job, and your anxiety level would go down. But when neither fight, flight, or freeze is an appropriate response, you are left standing in a fearful situation with your alarm sounding and your heart racing.

Now that you understand what is happening to your body, you can move on to the next step which will build on your ability to rate your anxiety and understand what is happening to your body.

WHEN ANXIOUS, STEP 3 IS TO FACE THE ANXIETY

Randomness is a terrible thing.

The most important step in reducing your anxiety is Step Three. When I teach it in therapy, I usually try to teach it in a session without Step Four to be sure that my client doesn't just skip over it and go on to the next. The temptation to skip it can be high, as you'll be doing the very thing that you have avoided for so long—facing your fear.

Let's take a step back from this process for a moment, and I want you to think about a typical thriller movie. Most thrillers have a similar format, with the first part of the film consisting of the protagonist running away from a monster or a threat. The more he runs, the stronger the threat becomes. No matter what he tries, the monster just keeps rearing its ugly head and attacking. Then at some point, exhausted and angry, the protagonist stops running and turns to face it. "Come on out," he yells, shining a flashlight in the monster's direction. It is at this point that the plot shifts, and the power transfers from the threat to the protagonist. The monster is about to be taken down.

This is where you are. You've done enough running away from your fear. It's exhausting, depleting, and it doesn't work (if it did, I'd try to teach you how to run faster). But the more you run, the greater your anxiety becomes. You might escape it for a moment or a day, but it will keep coming back until you decide to shine a flashlight on it.

For many people this sounds like an impossible task, and it wouldn't be unusual for you to have thoughts such as "I'll never be able to do this. I'm too afraid to try." But I want you to know that you can. Learning and practicing the following techniques will help get you there.

Here is a step-by-step guide on how to face anxiety:

- When you notice your anxiety increasing, try to take a curious and interested attitude instead of a judgmental one. Rather than, "Oh no this is bad. Why do I have this anxiety? What's wrong with me?" say to yourself, "Isn't that interesting that my anxiety is coming up in this situation."
- Then rate the anxiety using your scale. "I think this is a number ...."
- Know that you are not trying to stop the anxiety at this point. Trying to stop it is like trying to stop the rain from falling. Just like the changes in the weather, feelings come and feelings go. The anxiety can't last forever. It will move out on its own.
- Now say to yourself, "It's okay; it's just my anxiety. My body is going into fight, flight, freeze. It thinks there's a bear," and "My body thinks it's helping me."
- Then focus on specific areas of your body and connect them with what you now know about fight, flight, freeze. For example:

> Heart. If your heart is racing, focus on the feeling of it quickly beating. Move your consciousness into the feeling rather than away from it. Your heart can't make you do anything strange, it doesn't control your movements or words, it's just a quickly beating heart. Be kind to yourself. Think statements such as, "It makes sense that my heart is racing, something triggered my response and my heart is pumping blood throughout my body for energy."

Muscles. If you find that your muscles are getting tense, then focus on them. Is it mainly your arms or legs? Which part of your legs? Remind yourself, "It makes sense that my muscles are tight, my body is preparing to fight, run, or to stay in one position to hide. It doesn't know I can't hit the person in charge of this meeting."

Stomach. Your stomach might feel queasy. Focus on it. Does it feel tight or like butterflies? Connect this feeling with the fight, flight, freeze response. "This makes sense as my digestion has shut down."

- Practice sitting with your anxiety for extended periods. You can start with a few seconds or minutes. It doesn't matter where you begin. The most important thing is to increase your ability to sit with your feelings for longer periods of time.
- Some clients find it helpful to use a visualization technique while sitting with their anxiety. You can do this with your eyes open or closed.

    Imagine yourself sitting on a mountain watching a storm move in. You see the clouds starting to turn dark and heavy, and the rain beginning to fall. You feel the wind getting stronger and notice the sound of the leaves around you.
    You don't have to run away or protect yourself. Weather comes and weather goes, it can't last forever. There is nothing you need to do to make it go away. Just sit and watch. Still. It's starting to rain harder now, and you imagine yourself in the very center of the storm. It's raging all around you.
    You might feel claustrophobic. You might feel like you want to get out. It's not a pleasant feeling sitting here in the middle, but that's okay. You can still sit and watch. You are safe. You are strong. You have the courage to stay. It's taken a lot of strength to go through life with so much anxiety; you can use the same strength now. You can stay in the center observing for a while.

Then when you're ready, imagine yourself sitting at the top of the mountain. The rain is gone and the air smells fresh. The sky above you is clear and blue. You look down at the valley and you see the storm far below. It looks small from where you are. Distant. You watch as the clouds begin to break up and drift away.

- You will notice significant improvement if you start to think of your anxiety as something that you would like to have so that you can practice facing it. Perhaps you can even say to yourself, "I hope I have lots of anxiety this week so I can practice my steps."
- Practice every day. Practice alone. Practice with others. Practice on the way to events and on the way back. Practice. Practice. Practice. You will get better. And when you have mastered Step Three, you can move on to the next.

WHEN ANXIOUS, STEP 4 IS TO REDUCE THE ANXIETY

All the unknown freaks me out.

Hopefully by now you have discovered that the monster that's been chasing you is not as persistent as you thought it was. It might show up to bother you for a while, but then it has to go. It can't control your actions and you're getting better at not running away from it. In fact, you might even ask it to show up sometimes so that you can practice. And now that you are standing over it shining a flashlight in its face, it's time to take it down.

A word of warning before moving on to Step Four: - If by any chance you have not practiced Step Three enough to develop some mastery, please go back and practice some more. It's hard to take control of something when you are afraid and running away. You want the monster right next to you, in your line of sight. Only then can you conquer it.

All of the methods in the following rules work differently. Some give the body appropriate ways to fight, flight, or freeze, while others change your thinking or actually turn the alarm off. It's usually difficult to predict which method will work best for a person, so try them all. Sometimes you will only need to do one technique, at other times you will need to combine them.

If you are working with a child, practice each of the techniques and make a list of them on a sheet of paper. Next to the technique have the child draw a picture to remind her what it is. When she is anxious and it is time for Step Four, point to the paper (or a photo of it on your phone) and say, "Which one would you like to do for your anxiety?" Then guide her through the chosen technique by modeling and encouraging her. I have assigned some of the methods with a kid-friendly title which can also be used with adults.

If you are working with a child who is one of the more visual thinkers, she might enjoy making a movie of the different techniques. The more creative you can be with this the better, such as developing characters or saying "action." She can then watch herself doing the things she needs to do to calm down, and she might even replay it in her head when anxious.

REDUCE ANXIETY IN STEP 4
BY BREATHING DIAPHRAGMATICALLY

How it works: Turns off the fight or flight alarm by decreasing the heart rate. Helps the body to be still and quiet.
Effectiveness: Very effective.
Challenge: Using it when anxiety is over a 7 on the 10-point scale.
Technique name for children: Darth Vader Breath

Many people are told to "take a deep breath" when anxious, but they find it doesn't work. I want you to go ahead and take a few deep breaths right now. Do your shoulders or upper chest go up? Are you breathing through your nose? Are your breaths rapid, short, or choppy? If you answered "Yes" to any of these questions, then the reason it doesn't work is because you have been doing the deep breathing wrong. You've been doing the kind of breathing that

Strengthen Your Social Radar

keeps the anxiety alarm on and is made to increase the heart rate and quickly circulate oxygen throughout the body. It is the kind of breathing that gets you ready for action.

Just as one breath prepares your body for danger, there is another that will tell your body to relax, and will actually turn the alarm off. It does this by slowing your heart rate. When your heart is beating slowly, it's hard for your body to be in the anxiety mode. And the good news is that you can control how fast your heart beats.

Start by saying the word "her" but make it sound like Darth Vader or a scuba diver. It should come from the bottom of your throat. Next focus on using your stomach muscles to pull your stomach in (to look as skinny as you can) and out (I tell kids to try to look like Santa Clause). You can place your hand on your stomach as you practice moving your stomach in and out in slow, gentle movements. In traditional diaphragmatic breathing, the stomach movements are reversed so that when you breathe out you pull your stomach in. However, my clients find it simpler not to do this, and they still have excellent results, so we will learn without the reversal.

Therefore, make the "her" sound as you breathe out and push your stomach out. Breathe through your open mouth, not through your nose, making the Darth Vader sound. Practice it several times until it starts to feel more natural. As you push your stomach out and breathe out, think of the word "out." This word will act as an anchor point when you are anxious and need to start doing the technique. "Out," and you push your stomach out.

After you have mastered breathing out, you will add breathing in. For this breath you just do the opposite. You pull your stomach in towards your backbone, and take a deep breath in through your mouth. Make the same Darth Vader sound, coming from the bottom of your throat. When you are doing this breath, your shoulders shouldn't be moving up and down. You can place your fingertips on your shoulders to check this while you are practicing.

Practicing the technique before you become anxious is essential. The breath can be done anywhere. You can do it sitting down, standing up, walking around, talking, or lying down. As you gain mastery, you can stop doing the Darth Vader sound, as this is just useful in the beginning to be sure that you are breathing from the right area. Always start with your anchor thought of "Out," and push your stomach out.

One of the wonderful things about this technique is that you'll know right away when it's working. You may notice your face is more relaxed, or you might yawn, stretch, or lean back on the sofa. You can also know it's working by measuring your heart rate before and after the breathing to see how much it has dropped. In other words, you will clearly see how easily you can control the engine that drives your anxiety.

REDUCE ANXIETY IN STEP 4 BY REWIRING YOUR BRAIN'S CIRCUITS

People tell me to listen, but my mind gets stuck on this one detail. It keeps running over the same scenario and I can't hear anything being said.

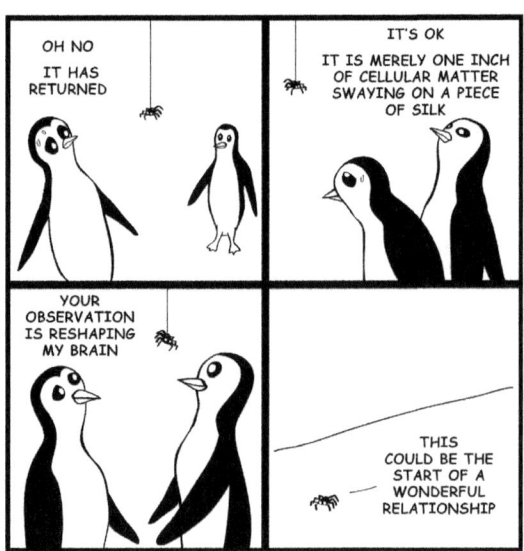

How it works: Alters the pathways of your brain cells.

Effectiveness: Children often start picking it up and using it after one session; adults can take longer.

Challenge: Remembering to practice, practice, practice — this is how the imprint of the new circuit is developed.

Technique name for children: *Oh no....... It's okay*

Obsessive thinking is a common characteristic of autism and can be very helpful when developing new ideas or areas of interest. But when the obsessive qualities are focused on anxious thoughts, they can quickly become destructive.

People can find themselves stuck in their fears, thinking the same things over and over. One client described it as feeling as though she was orbiting around a planet of terrible possibilities, unable to propel away. Another used the analogy of a sieve, where the holes were too small to allow his anxious thoughts to drop through.

These types of descriptions are common. Letting go of fears can be incredibly difficult, and this is made even more intense if you have a strong attention to detail. You might notice the bee buzzing in the corner, the storm clouds swirling, or the large noisy group about to enter the restaurant. When your mind gets stuck in a loop of fear, you end up in a place of negative and critical thoughts such as "I'll never be any good."

With children I call this place the *Oh No Land*. In sessions, I'll get a large piece of paper and draw a grumpy face with *Oh no* written underneath. We'll then go to *Oh No Land* by standing on the paper and verbalizing all of the thoughts and feelings you can have in it. "*Oh no...* the test is timed. *Oh no...* there's going to be a storm and I'm afraid my house will be destroyed. *Oh no...* I have to go somewhere new."

As with any pathway, whether it's a neural one in the brain or a trail in the woods, the more times you take the route, the stronger it becomes and the more likely it is that you will follow it.

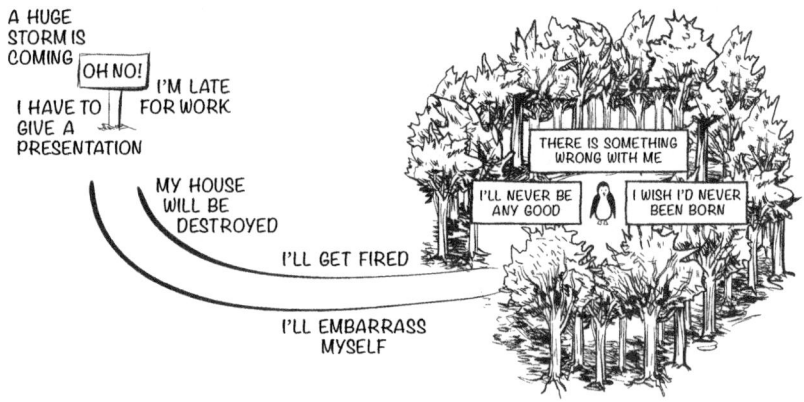

The good news about this neural pathway is that it can be changed. When you stop yourself from repeating these patterns of negative thinking, their connections in your mind will weaken. As the neural pathway starts to fade, you are less likely to follow it and end up in a place where you feel stuck.

You can develop a new pattern of thinking when a problem arises, something that will actually help you resolve the challenges you face. Studies have shown that when people change the way they think, it causes actual functional and structural changes in their brains. So, no matter what your age, you can rewire your mind and make it work better for you.

The first step in rewiring your brain is to develop an exit off the old pathway. You can't stop problems from arising, and you won't be able to get rid of all of the *Oh no* thoughts, as some of these will come from other people, but you can change where you go after this.

Instead of going down a long pathway of negative thoughts, I want you to insert a new thought after the *Oh no* appears in your mind. Start the new thought with the words *It's okay* and then challenge yourself to complete a sentence in your mind as to why it's okay. For example:

Oh no, my manager wants me to finish preparing the presentation in the next hour.
It's okay, I can use what I have and explain what I'd like to do for the future.

Oh no, I have to go to the office party.
It's okay, I went last year and got through it.

Oh no, I'm going to be late.
It's okay, everyone is late once in a while and I'm usually on time.

Oh no, the schedule has been changed.
It's okay, I can do my breathing as I walk to the new meeting.

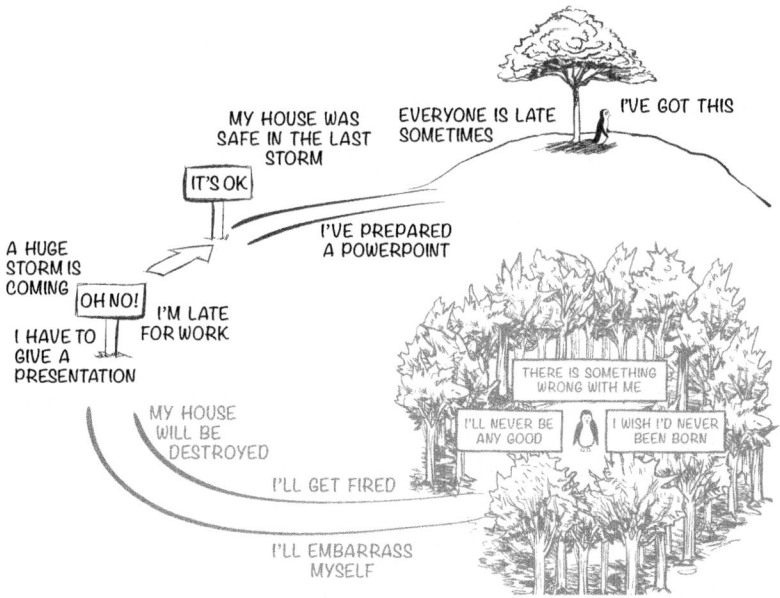

Be sure to start each sentence with the words *It's okay*, as these words will become a signal for your mind to go in the new direction. Then practice, practice, practice. It doesn't matter how you practice, but the more times you can make the *Oh no . . . It's okay* connection, the stronger and more automatic it will be become. To practice you can:

- Write down all the challenges you had in the day, and then write the *It's okay* statement under each one. This will also become a journal where you can monitor your progress.

- Don't worry if you don't feel immediately different after making the *It's okay* statement. When you rewire your brain, you are changing your thoughts first, and after a while your new thoughts will change your feelings.
- As soon as you recognize that your mind has gone onto the negative path, develop the *It's okay* thought. This may happen in the middle of the difficulty, or it might happen later in the day when you're thinking about it.
- Try to recognize when other people are having an *Oh no* moment, and then develop an *It's okay* thought that you could use if you are ever in the same situation.
- When I first teach it to a child, I will place a second piece of paper on the floor next to the *Oh no* one, and I'll write *It's okay* on it and draw a smiley face. I will then tell her to stand on the *Oh no* paper, and I'll call out a problem using the first-person point of view. "*Oh no*, the teacher asked for my homework and I left it in my backpack...." If the child can think of an *It's okay* she then calls it out and jumps to the other paper. "*It's okay*, I can ask the teacher if I can go and get it." The child gets one point if she can think of a new thought, and I get one point if she can't. I'll always give her some extra help if she needs it and reinforce how good she is at finding solutions to problems.
- Give children challenges throughout the day. Include the whole family and try to make it fun. "It's dessert time, I'll give you each an *Oh no*, and as soon as you think of an *It's okay* I'll scoop out your ice cream."

Just as walking along the same trail in the woods will make it clearer over time, practicing the different pattern of thinking will strengthen the new imprint in your brain. This new pathway of neurons will lead to finding solutions, to thinking creatively, and to feeling confident about your ability to get through challenges.

REDUCE ANXIETY IN STEP 4
WITH EXERCISE

My brain is like a whole bunch of TVs on the wall; they all come up in an instance making me feel anxious.

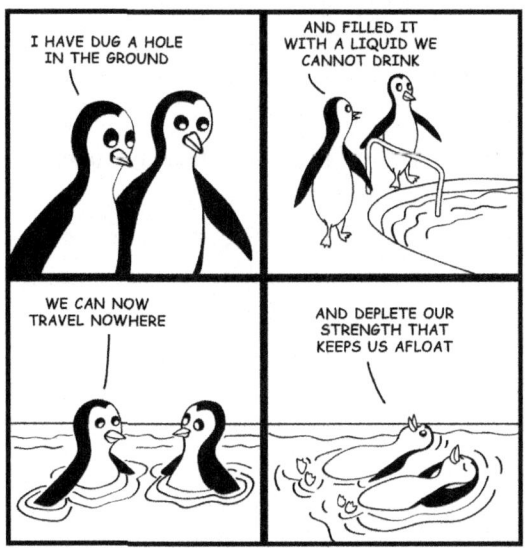

How it works: Releases chemicals called endorphins that improve mood, sleep, and tension. Distracts the mind from worries.

Effectiveness: An excellent technique to use in combination with other methods.

Challenge: Getting started and finding something that you enjoy.

The research is very clear; exercise is an effective tool for reducing anxiety. It allows your body to experience the same movements of fight or flight such as lifting, pushing, pulling, and running. It produces feel-good chemicals in your brain, and it gives sensory input of repetition and rhythm, all while providing a break from the stress of daily life.

Unfortunately, for the majority of the people I work with on the spectrum, exercise comes with unique challenges. This usually starts in elementary school

PE where the neurodiverse mind can be especially sensitive to the sounds of whistles, squeaky shoes on the gym floors, shouting, fast movement, and echoes. People on the spectrum often view balls as projectiles that hurt and decide that the best strategy is to get out of the way rather than to catch it and throw it back. And for clients who find reading social cues difficult, teammates can be especially hard to understand. All of this can result in teasing from peers and being the last one chosen for a team.

Finding the right exercise is key, and while everyone is different, there are some activities that can be a better fit. These are generally activities that require little reading of social cues, where balls are either absent or heading away from the person, and where movement is organized or rhythmic.

Examples include swimming, walking, hiking in nature, biking, martial arts, archery, rowing, and golf. If it's difficult to get motivated, start by doing these activities in shorter sessions until the habit is in place, and then slowly increase the amount of time.

REDUCE ANXIETY IN STEP 4 BY CHALLENGING IRRATIONAL FEARS

I was preparing myself for something bad to happen, but then I realized there was nothing to prepare for.

How it works: Challenges any lies that you have come to believe and replaces them with truth.
Effectiveness: Very effective.
Challenge: Accepting that your thoughts will need to change before your feelings can change.
Technique name for children: Be a Detective

It is likely that many of your fears are not based in reality, but come from events that happened in your life and from things that have happened to someone else. For example, you might have experienced an argument at a family reunion and developed a fear that all family gatherings will have conflict. Or perhaps you heard that someone's home was destroyed by a tornado, and you are now afraid that your own home will be destroyed.

These types of fears can become locked in your mind if you don't take some action to challenge them. Challenging the fear means holding it up against the likelihood that it will happen. Does the thing that you are afraid of happen to you frequently? Is it happening to people who live in circumstances similar to yours? Or is it a lie that you have come to believe?

To challenge your thoughts, make a chart with four columns. In the first column, write a prediction or fear — something disastrous that you worry will happen. For example: "I predict that my house will be destroyed in the storm" or "I predict that my uncle will shout at me at the family gathering." Try to be as specific as possible, and avoid generalities such as "the storm will be bad," or "I won't have a good time at the dinner." We need to know what "bad" or "a good time" actually look like.

In the following chart, we are using the example of a young woman with autism who was afraid of failing out of college. This is a fear that I have seen in several of my clients, especially those who feel very passionate about their studies. Because of her anxiety, she was avoiding doing her work. She thought it would not be good enough, even though she was a very high-achieving, intelligent student.

Her fear of failing led her to adopt other fears, such as a fear of being homeless due to low grades and a fear of losing the approval of her friends and family. She was about to have a math exam and was afraid that she would fail. As failure can look different depending on your goals, she defined it as a grade C or less.

She wrote her fears down in the first column under "Prediction/Fear" and completed the column on how this would make her feel.

PREDICTION / FEAR	I PREDICT I WILL FEEL	WAS I CORRECT?	ACTUAL OUTCOME
I will make a C or less on my math exam.	SAD		
When I make a C my family and friends will disown me.	SAD		

After the event has occurred, look at the chart and see if your prediction came true. If your fear/ prediction was not accurate, write "no" in the third column and put what happened in the "Actual Outcome" column. For this student, her outcome was an A on her math exam.

PREDICTION / FEAR	I PREDICT I WILL FEEL	WAS I CORRECT?	ACTUAL OUTCOME
I will make a C or less on my math exam.	SAD	NO	Happy I made an A
When I make a C my family and friends will disown me.	SAD	NO	Happy I made an A

Continue using the chart, writing down what you predict will happen. Then review its accuracy, correcting it if needed once you know the outcome. Most of my clients turn out to be wrong about their predictions. They don't fail their quizzes, midterms, or papers. Their houses aren't destroyed by tornadoes.

You will likely have a similar experience and develop a long list of inaccurate predictions. You will begin to realize that you are not very good at making predictions and that your fears are irrational. At this point, you will change your irrational belief to a rational one. For a student who has never made a C, it is irrational to be overwhelmed by a fear of failing.

PREDICTION / FEAR	I PREDICT I WILL FEEL	WAS I CORRECT?	ACTUAL OUTCOME
I will make a C or less on my math exam.	SAD	NO	Happy I made an A
When I make a C my family and friends will disown me.	SAD	NO	Happy I made an A
I will make a C on my midterm.	SAD	NO	Happy I made an A
I will make a B on my quiz.	HAPPY	NO	Happy I made an A
I will make a B on my exam.	HAPPY	NO	Happy I made an A
I will make an A on my exam.	HAPPY	YES	
I will make an A on my paper.	HAPPY	YES	

When working with a child who is challenging her fears, it's helpful to first explain the idea of prediction, and then ask if she is willing to investigate the topic she is worried about. Write her job title at the top of the chart. For example, write "Storm Detective" or "Academic Researcher." Explain that you need her help to find out more information. Perhaps the exams in her school are very difficult or storms are often destroying houses in her neighborhood.

Encourage her to write her predictions down each day. When you hear her make a prediction ("I know I'm going to fail this test!") point it out to her ("That sounds like a prediction") and have her write it on the sheet. Then, when she is ready to change her irrational fear to avoid another wrong prediction, explain that she is just writing down what she thinks even though she might still feel as if she is going to fail.

REDUCE ANXIETY IN STEP 4
WITH PROGRESSIVE MUSCLE RELAXATION

I can't eat with my family because the sight of the food will terrify me that I'll hear a chewing sound.

How it works: Makes the body feel as though it just completed fight, flight, or freeze.
Effectiveness: Very effective.
Challenge: Taking the time to practice even when you are not anxious.
Technique name for children: Squeeze and Stretch

One of the difficulties of fight, flight, or freeze is that everything in your body is preparing you to hit someone, run away, or to stay in a frozen position. With progressive muscle relaxation, you are giving your body the tight muscles it would expect if you were responding to danger, followed by the relaxed muscles you would normally have after the event. This makes your body feel as though the fight, flight, or freeze is finished, and it can turn your internal alarm off.

As muscle relaxation involves tightening and relaxing different muscles in your body, it also helps you become more alert to the differences between the anxious and relaxed states. You will be quicker at recognizing when your anxiety is setting in and better at knowing how to cue yourself out of it.

To practice this technique, begin by making two tight fists with your hands by your sides. Squeeze the fists as hard as you can without hurting yourself for about five seconds. Focus on what your fists feel like when tense; try not to tense other muscles such as your arms or shoulders in the process.

Open up your hands and allow your muscles to relax for fifteen seconds. Feel the tension flowing out of your fingertips, away from you. Notice the difference between the tense state and the relaxed state. One is tight and closed, the other is loose and open. Focus on this contrast.

You can then continue to tense and relax other muscles groups in your body. Try to practice daily, even if it's only in small amounts such as tightening and relaxing your hands when you are sitting at a red light. If you have racing thoughts at night this is a wonderful technique to do before sleeping.

The more you practice, the better prepared you will be to use this method when anxious. There are several different muscle groups you can tighten including:

> Feet: curl your toes under and squeeze.
>
> Legs: tighten calf and thigh muscles.
>
> Arms: tighten the bicep muscles by bending both arms at the elbow and release, then tighten the triceps by extending your arms out.
>
> Hands: close both hands into fists.
>
> Stomach and Chest: breathe in deeply and hold for four seconds.
>
> Shoulders: bring your shoulders up to your ears and tense the muscles.
>
> Mouth: open your mouth wide.
>
> Forehead: raise your eyebrows.
>
> Whole Body: bring your arms and legs into your body and squeeze.

If you are sensitive to certain sounds (common trigger sounds include eating, drinking, sniffing, whispering), learning to relax your muscles can help reduce feelings of anxiety and frustration. This is because hearing the sound will trigger a physical tension in the body, which will then trigger the negative feelings. When you hear the sound, try to become aware of which part of your body becomes tense. Then work on relaxing this muscle group when you are triggered.

When teaching children muscle relaxation, it will be important to keep things fun while showing them how to do the technique. For example, you can encourage them to relax into silly body positions and facial expressions, or stretch out as far as they can. You can also remind them that they can tighten their hands under their desk or by their sides when in class, and that they can usually curl their toes without anyone noticing.

REDUCE ANXIETY IN STEP 4
BY GOING BACK TO YOUR SENSES

*When people are gathered around me, I'm
scared they'll think I'm annoying.*

How it works: Takes you out of anxious thoughts and anchors your mind in the world around you.
Effectiveness: Can be very effective in a variety of different settings.
Challenge: Harder when you are feeling tired or when the anxiety stems from physical pain or illness.
Technique name for children: 5...4...3...2...1

Getting back to your senses directs the mind onto a new course by interrupting the replaying of worries and fears. It grounds you in the present and helps you to feel centered. The technique is simple and can be repeated as many times as you need. Out loud or in your mind, name:

> 5 things you can currently see.
>> They can be large things like a tree, or as small as a dot on a table. It doesn't matter as long as you can see it.
>
> 4 things you can hear.
>> Name any external sounds, not thoughts in your mind.
>
> 3 things you can feel.
>> If you want to, you can move around and feel things in the environment.
>
> 2 things you can smell.
>
> 1 thing you can taste.

TURN THE ANXIETY DOWN BY LEARNING WHAT *NOT* TO DO

It takes more energy for me to be in social settings.

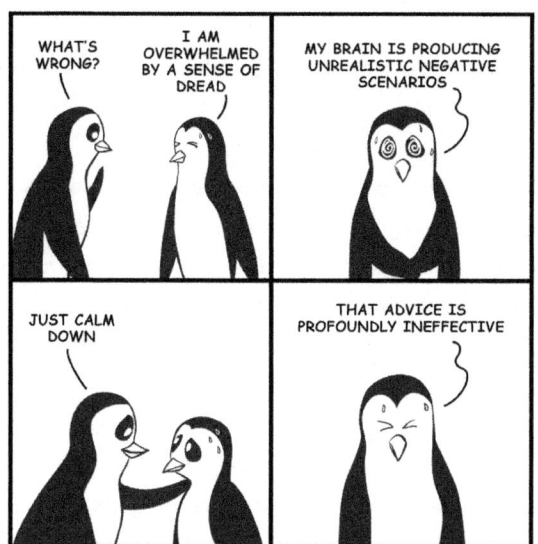

For some of my clients who receive a diagnosis of autism later in life or who have had little access to treatment, levels of anxiety can be very high. Meeting new people, being in social groups, and managing sensory information is often overwhelming when you don't understand the reason for your difficulties, or you have limited coping skills. It is understandable that people in these situations will look for any means to relieve their stress, even unproductive ones. Unfortunately, a common strategy is to self-medicate with drugs or alcohol.

Substance use can dull sensory information and reduce the noise of the social world, making the person feel more relaxed and confident. Drugs and alcohol also provide an instant social group, whether it's the kids who are smoking or vaping marijuana at school or the adults getting together in a bar, there is a predictable place and pattern to using that can be comforting. In these situations, the focus is on the substance use more than the social interactions, differences between people are more likely to be accepted, and buying someone a drink or sharing drugs can lead to instant new "friends."

If you have stepped into this world, it can feel like a great relief at first. You might experience sentiments of "At last I've found something that makes me feel good," "I feel important when I buy the alcohol," "I feel accepted," or "I finally feel like I can connect." However, when reliance is placed on the drug for these feelings, you are not doing what you need to do to address the underlying needs of building social skills, managing anxiety, and making real connections.

Just like other substance users, you might have gone so far into your addiction that you are struggling to get out, and it is especially challenging for someone on the spectrum to stop using due to some unique factors. Difficulties in reading social cues make it hard to discern if other people embedded in the drug culture are using you for their own needs or if they are a true friend. When a drug dealer says, "Take this; it will make you feel better," or "I'm your friend so I'm going to give you some free drugs to help you," you might find it more difficult to identify if they are telling the truth. If a person lies about a friendship in order to have a free place to stay or access to your money, property, or physical self, it can be confusing. "Why would they do that if they don't care about me?" is a common question I'm asked by clients in this situation.

Becoming sober will have unique challenges. Traditional drug treatment of sharing experiences in a group setting can be overwhelming, and residential treatment centers may feel claustrophobic. The lack of social skills that was a factor leading into this problem becomes compounded with the difficulties of maintaining sobriety.

It is essential that any program of recovery is prepared to treat both the challenges of the substance use and the autism. There should be at least one staff member who understands autism and can educate the rest of the team. Programs should also include elements such as individual therapy, medication consultations, cognitive behavioral therapy, social skill training, family education, art therapy, music therapy, modeling, vocational training, outdoor activities, and a strong mentoring program.

DEVELOP AN EMERGENCY EXIT PLAN

When I'm anxious I don't feel socially alert.

Some social situations will still be challenging, even if you have followed all the rules and practiced reducing anxiety. You might be asked a question that you don't know how to answer, find yourself getting pulled into an argument, be caught in an overwhelmingly crowded or noisy place, or end up in a conversation with someone who makes you anxious.

It's during these stressful times that things can go quickly wrong, and the best course of action can be to leave the situation so that you can collect your thoughts, "cool off," or have a sensory break. An emergency exit consists of three elements — a stressor, an alarm, and an exit.

A stressor can be anything that will take you out of your normal balanced state and make you feel anxious, angry, or just highly uncomfortable. It might be a person, place, something sensory, or an unwanted event. Some common stressors include seeing someone whom you don't like, having unwanted attention, crowds, noise, an unexpected change in routine, people doing things the "wrong" way, or becoming involved in an argument. Learn to recognize the stressors that are making you want to leave so that you can become more aware of situations that are particularly challenging for you. Although you might not recognize the stressor in the moment, you will probably be able to identify it later on ("I know what made me angry; it was the ...").

When the challenging situation occurs, your internal alarm will go off. This alarm will increase your level of anxiety and the "fight, flight, freeze" response is activated. If you decide that for this situation you want to "flight," you will need to find an exit.

As anyone who has been on an airplane knows, the exits are pointed out before the journey begins, not in the middle of an emergency. The same needs to be true of your evacuation plan. Don't wait until you are in a difficult social situation to look for ways out. Identify them now. Then when you need to leave, all you need to do is choose which one you want to use.

The following chart shows examples of different exit strategies.

EXIT	WHEN TO USE	HOW TO USE
The Honest Exit	Best for family, friends, and people who accept you.	Just be honest, sharing as much as you want about the stressor, alarm, and need for an exit. For example: "I think I need to take a break. I'm just going outside for a few minutes, and then I'll be back." "All the noise and arguing is making me feel anxious. I'm going for a walk to cool off, and then maybe we can talk about it when I get back."
The Instant Exit	When you don't want anyone to know that you're feeling uncomfortable and you need to leave immediately.	Take your phone out of your pocket, and quickly look at your recent call log. Then, with your phone still in your hand, say, "I'm sorry, I'll be right back," and step outside. Use the time to text or call a friend, and then return when you're ready.
The Helpful Exit	When you're not too annoyed or anxious, but you're starting to feel uncomfortable and need to move to a different area.	Look for something you can help with, and use it as an excuse to move away from the person you're talking to. For example: "I'm going to get a coffee; can I get you one?" If the person says yes, bring him back a coffee and then move to a new area. Or say, "Excuse me, I'm just going to . . . help set up the chairs. . . . see if they need any help in the kitchen. . . . help with the outside activities.

EXIT	WHEN TO USE	HOW TO USE
The Bathroom Break	When you need a few minutes to shut everything out. This is especially useful if you have sensory overload.	Slip away to the bathroom. Just a few minutes behind a closed door or bathroom stall can help you recover. Don't be longer than 10 minutes.

If you're in a public building with several bathrooms, choose a bathroom a little further away from the event such as a bathroom on a different floor. The short walk will help you calm down, and you'll be less likely to see people you know in there.

During the break you can wash your hands to literally cool down. |
| The Cavalry Call | Good when you're in a difficult situation and your social guide is with you. | Arrange with your social guide that you will text him a code word such as "Thanks," when you need his help. Keep the code word inconspicuous rather than "SOS. Come get me!!!!" just in case someone sees the text.

Have your social guide wait about 5 minutes then come get you. The wait is so that the person you're talking to doesn't see you send a text and then immediately see your friend come rushing over with a concerned look on his face.

Your friend can casually join the conversation and then lead you away. Or they can do a more direct, "Excuse me, I just need you for a moment." You can then look very sorry to leave the conversation. |

AUTISM RULES

EXIT	WHEN TO USE	HOW TO USE
The Mind-Only Exit	When your body has to stay, but your mind needs to leave. Good for situations where you do not need to be actively talking to others or paying attention to every detail.	This is called dissociation or detachment. It's a way to protect yourself against unwanted feelings, and if used every day, it can be considered unhealthy. But if it's used occasionally, it can be an excellent exit strategy. Mild detachment: My clients have discovered several creative activities to do in their minds including counting numbers, playing with numbers, playing music in their heads, listing information, listing names, visualizing their schedules. Mild detachment can also include doodling and daydreaming. Moderate Detachment: Playing a movie in your mind that you like or recently saw, playing a video game in your mind, playing back a memory that you liked. Good for situations where you have a sensory overload, such as stuck on a hot school bus and everyone is singing a song you don't like. With moderate detachment you will not be talking to anyone or taking notes. Be aware that when you are playing a video in your mind, and someone in your environment talks to you, the interruption may feel like a glitch in your video streaming.

SOME MAPS CAN GET YOU LOST

My autism makes it easier for me to pick up on patterns, long and complex.

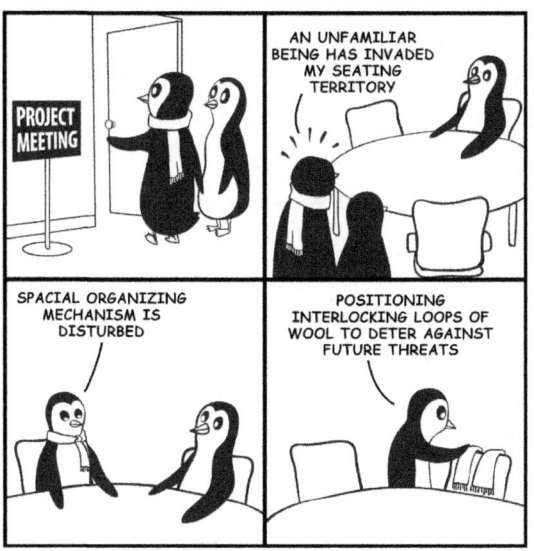

When neurotypicals think about maps, they usually just imagine a digital GPS or an old-fashioned paper map. But for many autistic people, mapping is a much more creative and diverse process. It can involve studying maps and recreating them from memory or visualizing maps of shopping centers with details of each store. These skills are very helpful if you want to find something quickly or restock shelves. It's the same technique that engineers use when figuring out how to fit the pieces of a machine together or identify parts that are out of place.

This mapping often goes beyond geographic locations to include maps of numbers, time, and social situations. Numbers can be assigned to a variety of people and things such as peers in a class, license plates, and significant dates. They can be organized on a large chart and studied for interesting patterns. When mapping time, many of my clients imagine a long line in their minds with different points representing the expected events of their day. They then follow the map from point to point as each event occurs.

With social situations, there can be a variety of different maps. A college student who was having difficulty communicating described that when a person spoke to him, he would map out all the possible ways of replying, taking into consideration how his past responses have succeeded or failed. It was like a giant flow chart in his mind that was constantly searching for information as the conversation shifted. Another client shared how she has a map in her mind where everyone sits for her office meetings.

The problem with all this mapping is that it can get you lost. Not physically lost as when you can't find your way home, but psychologically. This usually happens in two ways: The first is when you become overly dependent on using maps and you find yourself in a situation without one. The second is when the map you have doesn't fit the reality. Both of these situations can leave you feeling as if something is "wrong" with the world around you. The word "some" is included in the title of this rule because what I don't want you to do is throw out the whole concept of mapping. It's an excellent skill, and if used in the right way can be a great strength. Here are some guidelines on how to use mapping in a way that strengthens your social radar.

- Accept "recalculating" as a normal part of mapping. Don't become attached to your map to the point where you view it as a fixed, rigid representation of reality. Instead, think of it as an adjustable map which must be revised to reflect reality. Some parties will be canceled at the last moment. A store will alter its layout. Your peers in the class will line up in a different order. Don't get pulled into thinking that these changes are wrong. Rather, say to yourself "recalculating" and alter your map to fit the new circumstances. If you are a parent, you can have your child look at your GPS as you are driving, and show them how it recalculates when you take different turns. "I think I want to go this way as there are less cars. Look at the map recalculating. The rule is a good map will quickly recalculate when things change. Can you recalculate the map in your mind too?"

- Be aware that keeping maps open in your brain will drain your mental energy. It can be a burden to constantly worry about constructing and comparing your map. Practice relying on the other social skills taught in this section, along with the 5Ws of conversation. You will develop useful intuitions and exhaust less mental energy.
- Practice using other skills when orienting yourself in a location. You can then develop flexibility by switching between the skills below and using mental maps. Examples of skills include:

  > Think of getting lost as part of the adventure. You might see something interesting in a department you wouldn't normally explore or gain a new perspective by entering a different area. Understand that most people approach activities like shopping this way, and you'll be less frustrated when you see your friends and family wandering around in stores for long periods of time.

  > Look for written signs that offer directions. If the sign is different to what you had in your mind be open to recalculating your map.

  > Ask staff where something is located. Use this as an opportunity to gather more information about what your visiting, such as the best time of day to avoid crowds.

  > Get subtle clues from other people. What are they carrying? ("A lot of people have coffee, so I must be near the cafe!") What direction are they coming from?

  > Challenge yourself by going to places that you haven't mentally mapped out. Choose environments that will still be safe if you get lost.

REMEMBER TO ASK YOURSELF, "WHAT ARE THEIR FEELINGS UP TO?"

My friends are upset that I don't want to FaceTime them. Why would I want to FaceTime anyone? I already know what people's faces look like.

When I was in a creative writing class, I was advised to tape a piece of paper on the wall saying, "What are the other people up to?" This was to remind me that while I was paying attention to the hero's storyline, other characters were also busy doing something. It was important that I didn't forget their stories, and that I took some time to write about them too.

In the same way, it can be easy to get caught up in your own storyline or feelings. It might be that you're talking about something you're passionate about, learning about a new interest, or explaining your point of view, and in your excitement, you forget to think about how the people around you are feeling.

Identifying people's feelings can be difficult. It's very common for someone on the spectrum to fail to recognize that the person he is talking to is experiencing boredom or irritation, but if you can remember to think about the other person's feelings, your social radar is immediately strengthened. And when you can't figure out what the person is feeling, you can always ask.

You can be open and direct with those who know you and accept you. For example, "Am I boring you? I may be having an autism moment and talking too much about this." You can also be more indirect for those who do not know you as well, "I'm wondering if there's something else you wanted to do today. We could ..." or "I'm wondering if you might be feeling differently about this."

Like the piece of paper on my wall, you will need to put a note in your mind or on your phone that reminds you to ask yourself, "What are their feelings up to?"

FIRST EASY, THEN DIFFICULT

*I like to learn one thing and then optimize it,
not learn new things every day.*

Just like an athlete doesn't wait until the day of the Olympics to practice a difficult move, you shouldn't wait until you're in a demanding social situation to get better at your skills.

New ways of doing things should be practiced in the least demanding social situations where it doesn't matter too much if you fail. For example, practicing sending a text to your social guide to help you exit a situation would be better practiced at a public event where you don't know anyone, rather than at your office talking to your boss.

When working with a child, it will be particularly important to plan practice sessions that first meet the criteria of the easy category. This will help in building confidence while keeping anxiety low. Ask her to rate on a scale of ten how difficult she found the practice session. If her rating is above a seven switch to some easier situations for additional practice. You can then slowly move to more demanding situations.

In easy social situations:

- The cost of failure is low. It doesn't matter too much if things go wrong or if you have to stop in the middle and start again.
- You are role-playing situations. This is when you act out a potential scene so that you can practice a specific skill. You might be at home, in therapy, or with a friend. You can record yourself and then watch it or have a social guide give you feedback.
- You are in a situation with low visibility. Not many people see you practicing, and those who do see you are supportive, understanding, don't care too much what you are doing, don't know you, or won't ever see you again.

- You are emotionally calm. There are few stressors to send you into fight, flight, freeze or high anxiety.
- The practice session is scheduled. You prepared yourself for the practice. You knew in advance where you were going and what skill you were going to do.
- Those around you are less likely to catch your social mistakes (young children, people from a different culture who might also be learning the unwritten rules).
- You are working on a familiar skill that you have practiced before.
- You are using notes, visuals or a written script to help guide you.

In difficult social situations:

- The cost of failure is high. If it goes wrong, there will be a consequence such as a loss of job or reputation.
- It is a real-life situation. You only have one chance to get it right. You can't pause, discuss, rewind, or try again.
- You have high visibility. There are many people watching you, and some of these people may not understand or support you.
- You are emotionally charged. You are already in fight, flight, freeze or have high anxiety. This includes environments with bright lights, noise, or crowds.
- The practice session is unscheduled. You didn't know you were going to practice the skill. It came as a surprise and you are not prepared.
- Those around you have excellent social skills and may be critical of those who don't.
- You are working on a new skill. You are practicing the skill for the first time.
- You do not have any notes, visuals or written scripts to help guide you.

DON'T FORGET THE HAPPY ENDING

It's exhausting to see everything in a room.

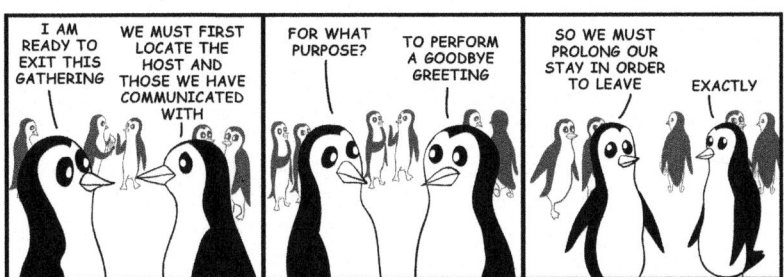

A good book or movie can be easily ruined by a poor ending, as it is the last thing in people's memories. As you develop your skills for a social event or work, you must not forget the last scene. Many of my clients put so much effort into managing all the social interactions during an event, that by the time it comes to leaving, they get up and go without saying goodbye. Their main concern at this point is getting out and getting home. Leaving an event is necessary, but doing it poorly is not.

For a happy ending, be careful not to leave too early or stay too long. You can follow the 'time to leave a party rule' in Chapter 2. Try to resist the temptation to do a "ghost goodbye," which involves slipping out without saying goodbye to anyone. People often view this as rude.

Then when you are ready to go, leave during a natural break, such as someone finishing a personal story, a change of speakers, applause, a coffee break, or a change of activities. Thank your host and give a genuine specific compliment about the event ("The chicken was delicious." "I really enjoyed the treasure hunt"). If you can't find a specific one, then give a vague compliment such as, "This was wonderful."

If you met someone you liked and you can remember his name, use his name when you leave. "It was great to meet you, Jim." Always look for the exit details of other people who are leaving. For example, did people take their leftover potluck food with them or leave it on a plate for others to finish?

AUTISM RULES

CHAPTER 4

Educate Others About How Your Mind Works

You might not realize how unique some of your skills are. When I ask people on the spectrum if they can visualize places they have visited or movies they have viewed, they will often reply, "Sure, I can see them really clearly" as though this is rather obvious. Then they'll tell me how they can watch a movie in their minds scene by scene, remember whole chunks of dialogue, describe the details of a place, or visualize all the scenes from a video game.

I'll ask, "Did you know that most people can't do this?"

"They can't?" they say, surprised.

One woman even closed her eyes and described all the small details of things in my office, many of which I haven't even noticed myself. Other clients taste certain foods more strongly or hear sounds more clearly. One young man became very quiet every time he went out with his girlfriend to crowded places. It wasn't until we discovered that he could hear all the conversations in the room at the same time, that we could work towards a solution. When his girlfriend asked why he hadn't mentioned it earlier he explained, " I thought that everyone could do that."

It can be hard to know what things about yourself are different from others. For this reason, you will often have a hard time educating people about how your mind works. This can lead to misunderstandings that are similar to the challenges people experience when two different cultures meet.

IT'S IMPORTANT TO EXPLAIN YOUR DIFFERENCES TO OTHERS

I constantly cried as a child because people didn't understand me.

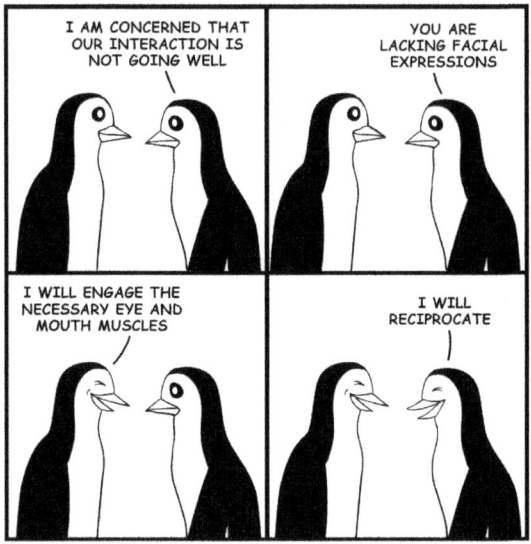

If the neurotypical culture understands how you think and feel, they can adjust to meet your needs. For example, one employee left a job because he "couldn't cope with the work environment." If he'd just told his supervisor the ticking clock annoyed him, his boss might have replaced it with a digital one.

In this chapter, I've tried to make it easier for you to communicate the differences by including a list of traits that are specific to people who are on the spectrum. As you read the list, check the box of any trait that applies to you. If you want feedback from others, you can hand the list to a friend, family member, teacher, or work colleague who can check the items that describe you. These will be your rules — Your way of thinking and feeling.

Under each trait, you will see examples of how certain traits can be used as a strength and how other people can help you. It might be that they can adjust your responsibilities to focus more on your strengths, help you to adjust to the challenge, or teach you a new skill.

Each trait also has a space for notes where you can add personal details or examples. For example, under "I'm sensitive to sounds," you can list sounds that annoy you such as "ticking clocks." You can also add your own solutions, such as "digital clocks are great." Once you have completed the list, you can use it to educate others about how your mind works. Different ways you might use the list include:

- Helping you realize how you are different from other people. If something is on the list, then most people do not feel or act this way.
- Handing the list to the people you interact with such as a spouse, boss, family member, career coach, teacher.
- Using it to develop goals to be included in an Individualized Educational Plan (IEP) at school or an Individualized Plan for Employment (IPE).
- Memorizing the traits so that you can explain the differences to others.
- Using the list to identify areas of strengths.
- For parents, look at the items and see which ones apply to your child. This will help you understand your child and be better equipped to meet his or her needs.

IDENTIFY THE TRAITS OF YOUR SPECTRUM MIND

☐ Check this box when the item describes you.
→ The arrow gives a little more detail on an item and an example of how people can help you with this trait.
+ The plus shows how this quality can be used as a strength.
_ You can add your notes in the space below each trait.

SOCIAL

I'm sorry I do not align with your social standards.

- ☐ My facial expressions are sometimes flat or not expressive. For example, I might not be smiling when I'm happy or excited.
- → Be careful not to interpret my blankness as negativity. Just say, "I'm not sure what you're feeling about this. Can you tell me?" Encourage me to develop my facial expressions through speech therapy, counseling, and group therapy.
- + The ability to keep my competition guessing can be useful in some situations.

_____

_____

- ☐ I avoid eye contact or look away from the person I am talking to.
- → Remind me to look in your direction when you are talking. If I look at your ear it will seem as if I'm looking in your eyes, and it can be less painful for me. Talk to me with your back turned towards me and explain that how I am feeling talking to your back is how neurotypicals feel when I don't make eye contact. Try filming me to help me understand how I appear to others.
- + I can be paying attention even though I'm not looking at you.

_____

_____

Educate Others

- ☐ Working in groups is difficult.
- → Don't put me in charge of managing people or organizing the timeline for a project. If I'm offered a promotion that involves managing people, it might be better for me to decline it. When working in groups, give me a specific and well-defined task that uses my skills, while allowing me to work independently. I can then bring my specific piece back to the group.
- \+ I'm good at generating my own ideas.

_____

_____

- ☐ I'm unaware of many social rules.
- → If I'm breaking a social rule or doing something that looks strange, please tell me. I probably didn't know I'm breaking an unwritten rule.
- \+ The unconventional often brings creative change.

_____

_____

- ☐ I appear to lack empathy.
- → Tell me directly how you feel and what I can do. Develop my ability to show empathy through concrete situations (if you step in a puddle I can see that your pants are muddy and I can practice helping). Teach me the rule on cognitive caring.
- \+ I care deeply about things I understand and am interested in.

_____

_____

- ☐ I react differently to physical closeness. I might not like being hugged, or I might sit and stand too close.
- → Rejecting your hug does not mean that I'm rejecting you; it's just that it feels uncomfortable for me. If I'm too close, tell me to move and remind me of any unwritten rules I am breaking. Keep the rules specific, such as "stand an arm's length away."
- + I might really appreciate hugs that I've initiated.

_____

_____

- ☐ I can overreact when distressed, angry, or anxious.
- → Don't just tell me to calm down or send me out of the room to calm myself down. This is like sending a person with Dyslexia to his room to learn to read. Instead, teach me how to be calm by showing me what to do. Use the techniques from the rules on how to turn the anxiety down. When angry, I can take a walk, listen to music, hit a punching bag, run, read, deep breathe, draw, kick a soccer ball, play basketball, spend time with my interests.
- + You will know when something has upset me.

_____

_____

- ☐ As a child, it's hard for me to get along with others my own age. As an adult, it can be difficult for me to connect with my own children.
- → Children are noisy, unpredictable, rule breakers, and difficult to anticipate, all very stressful qualities. I'll be better at connecting with children when engaged in a common interest that we both enjoy. More structured activities will be easier. You can structure them by setting a time limit,

Educate Others

clarifying rules and expectations, making a schedule, and having fewer participants.
+ As a child, I can be great with younger children and adults.

_____

_____

☐ I like to make maps of things like locations, numbers, conversations, and other patterns. I can keep these in my mind and use them in different situations.
→ Help me to communicate to you what I am mapping. Teach me other skills to use in those situations by using the techniques from the mapping rule.
+ I can be excellent at geographical orientation, finding mathematical patterns, and noting differences in patterns.

_____

_____

☐ When stressed, my mind can feel like a shaken snow globe.
→ Be aware that if I have challenging social situations, unexpected events, or sensory overload my mind can feel chaotic and I can't perceive things clearly. Give me extended time alone for my thoughts to settle.
+ When I am in optimal conditions I can have excellent focus and processing.

_____

_____

- ☐ Sudden changes in a schedule, routine, or events are difficult. It is especially challenging if it is something that has been planned for a long time or if it involves the cancellation of an activity in my area of interest.
- → Give me as much advanced warning as possible and make the change visual by putting it on a calendar. When the change is immediate, warn me first that a change is coming so that I can calm myself down and then tell me what it is.
- + I love routine and have a high tolerance for repetition.

_____

_____

- ☐ It's difficult for me to make friends
- → It's easier for me to make friends through activities, clubs, and common interests. Texting can be easier than phone calls. I can join a social skills group for people my own age to make friends and learn new skills.
- + I can be very loyal to the friends I have.

_____

_____

Educate Others

COMMUNICATION

*It's painful to have so much logic
in a world that lacks it.*

- ☐ It can be hard for me to have conversations.
- → Use other means of communication with me such as music, art, doing things together, or spending time in silence. Remind me not to just walk away when I'm finished talking. If I'm in school, enroll me in a lunch bunch group where I can have lunch with a small group of peers and practice conversation skills. Speech therapy can help with my pragmatic language skills.
- + Not everyone wants a lot of chatter.

_____

_____

- ☐ I take things literally.
- → Avoid vague language, metaphors, sarcasm, slang, hints, innuendos. Use concrete and specific language. If I don't get a joke, explain it to me. If you want something specific from me, tell me. If you use abstract language, immediately follow it with the concrete interpretation. "It's raining cats and dogs. It's really raining a lot."
- + If you say, "Work starts at 9:00," I will be walking through the door at 8:59.

_____

_____

- ☐ My voice sounds different from other people. It might have a different inflection, be monotone, sing-song, rapid, or sound like I'm speaking with the caps lock on.
- → Speech therapy can help my tone of voice.
- + I might be good at doing different character voices or acting roles where my voice is appreciated (Mr. Spock, Robots, Terminator, Castiel from Supernatural).

_____

_____

- ☐ I ask too many inappropriate questions.
- → If we are in a group and my questions are heading in the wrong direction, give me a nonverbal cue that only I will notice, or send me a reminder text. Later on, explain to me why it was inappropriate.
- + I ask the questions that everyone else wants to ask, but doesn't dare to.

_____

_____

- ☐ My language can sound like a professor, or I might repeat words or phrases out of context.
- → Speech therapy can help improve my language.
- + I can be good at remembering technical language.

_____

_____

Educate Others

- ☐ I don't ask for help when I need it.
- → Give me someone specific to go to for help. Set up a system where I am expected to ask questions. For example, tell me, "At our weekly review, please bring two questions that you have about your work." "I'd like you to ask one question in every math class." If I'm in college, encourage me to go to the professor's office hours during the first two weeks of class to establish a relationship.
- + I'm an independent worker.

_____

_____

- ☐ I talk too much about my own interests.
- → If we are in a social setting, give me a non-verbal sign that reminds me to use the index cards & 5Ws discussed in Chapter 2. You can help me be engaged in something by relating it to my interests.
- + Others will know what I like.

_____

_____

- ☐ I will often say what I think.
- → Remind me of the honest, kindness, and free speech rules in Chapter 2.
- + Every organization needs someone who will "tell the emperor when he has no clothes."

_____

_____

SENSORIMOTOR

Bad texture overrides a good flavor.

- ☐ I'm a picky eater.
- → Try not to mix foods together but serve them separately in military style. Avoid soups with unidentified floating objects. Know that changing the texture of a food (soft, crisp) can change the taste for me. Introduce new foods slowly with small amounts. Giving me a strong-tasting food that I like, such as mint, can help me cope with flavors I dislike. Iced water can help numb my taste buds.
- + A refined pallet makes me an excellent cook. I may want to cook so that I can prepare food the way I like it.

_____

_____

- ☐ I notice things that are out of place.
- → I might notice an object in the wrong container, a paint chip, crooked painting, or an editing error. I might like things to be lined up perfectly and become upset if you move them. Know that seeing these things not only distracts me but also makes me anxious. Place my desk away from distractions or give me a workspace with a divider. Let me know if I can rearrange something.
- + I can be excellent at noticing visual errors.

_____

_____

- ☐ I'm sensitive to bright lights.
- → Bright fluorescent lighting or sun can hurt my eyes. I might wake up earlier in the morning due to light in my room or feel uncomfortable in a classroom with fluorescent lights. Give me sunglasses to wear outside, provide me with sensory breaks, or change to halogen lighting. Use blackout curtains.
- + I enjoy watching flashing lights, patterns made by shadows, and things that sparkle, such as stars.

_____

_____

- ☐ I'm sensitive to sounds. Certain sounds startle me. I might feel disgusted or suddenly become angry at some sounds. It can be challenging for me to focus if I hear the sound.
- → It's not that I'm trying to be difficult, but I really do hear things better than most people. Annoying sounds can include ticking clocks, people chewing, people opening bags of food for their snacks, students talking in class, vacuum cleaners, loud echoes, whistles. If you want to know what it's like for me to be overwhelmed by sound, imagine trying to work while sitting next to a jackhammer on the highway. If a certain sound makes me angry, I might have misophonia. This causes me to feel disgust and have a fight or flight response. To help me, please remove the sounds, or allow me to use ear buds, earplugs, or noise-canceling headphones. Play music I like.
- + I can be skilled at technical repairs where I need to identify any changes in the sound of machinery. Good pitch discrimination.

_____

_____

- ☐ I'm sensitive to certain fabrics.
- → If I'm making a fuss about wearing certain clothes, it might just be because it's too tight, too itchy, or too stiff. Collars, socks with seams, and long pants can all be uncomfortable for me. Cut off tags in clothing. Turn clothes inside out so that the seam is on the outside. Look for soft fabrics and have me try items before purchasing them. A soft undershirt can help.
- + Soft blankets, soft clothes, and fitted undershirts can be calming.

_____

_____

- ☐ I react differently to touch.
- → Some tactile sensations can be very calming. Try the following to see which ones are helpful for me:

    Put several heavy blankets and/or coats over me when I'm in bed.
    Give me a soft blanket that I can wrap myself in.
    Gently squeeze my arm with one hand, starting at the top of the arm and working your way down to the fingers.
    Scratch my back or the inside of my arm with your nails, moving in one direction from top to bottom.
    As I lie down, put a pillow on my body. Then gently push on the pillow to apply pressure. Work from the top of the torso and arms, down to the legs and feet.
    Avoid unexpected and light touch.
    Give me a natural sponge to wash with.
    Have stress toys or textured objects available for me to feel.
- + An expected tight hug can be wonderful.

_____

_____

Educate Others

- ☐ I'm sensitive to smells.
- → Know that I really can smell things better than you, and it can be overwhelming or make me nauseous. Let me help you choose your perfume or aftershave if you want me to be close. If I like to seek out smells, remind me to have appropriate behavior in public and not sniff people or objects. Help me find a lotion, oil, or perfume that I like, and remind me to use it when other smells are too strong.
- + I can have excellent culinary and wine sommelier skills.

_____

_____

- ☐ I can be clumsy and uncoordinated.
- → I might knock into objects, bump into people, trip, or fall. Please know that my body does not experience the world the same way as yours and that I am not always aware of the position of my body. Get me some help from an occupational therapist. Don't force me into sports that I don't want to do if balls are coming towards me, such as football, soccer, or basketball.
- + Golf, archery, rowing, martial arts, and swimming are often good sports for me.

_____

_____

- ☐ I have a self-stimulating behavior such as pacing, rocking back and forth, flapping hands, or making sounds/ noises.
- → Encourage me to find a more socially-acceptable way to self-regulate, such as squeezing a stress ball, taking a break, using a swing or hammock,

swimming, taking a shower, raking leaves, digging, mowing the lawn, carrying heavy books, or going for a walk. Occupational therapy for sensory integration.
+ I wish you knew how wonderful stimming feels.

_____

_____

☐ I have poor handwriting and other fine motor skills.
→ Occupational therapy can help with this. If I'm a visual thinker, help me to notice the shapes and angles of the lines in handwriting. Try raised-lined writing paper and pencil grips. Let me try different pencils and pens to find one that feels good. Don't criticize my bad penmanship in front of the class.
+ I can be motivated to learn typing.

_____

_____

☐ I need alone time.
→ Processing sensory information and coping with social situations can be overwhelming, and I need time alone to feel balanced and to function effectively in the world around me. Understand that this is a neurological need and not because I don't value our time together.
+ Alone time is a simple thing to put in place.

_____

_____

COGNITIVE

My mind records things that I can't erase.
They suddenly come up and start playing.

- ☐ I know a lot about my area of interest.
- → Connect me with others who have similar interests through classes, conventions, clubs, internet groups. We all like to have some friends who are similar to ourselves. It will be easier to engage me in something if you can relate it to my area of interest. Allow me time to study my interest at the end of the day. Try to connect with me by talking about things I am interested in, and find something that you can like about it too (see the celebrate through play rule in Chapter 5).
- + I can be excellent in a career that matches my interest.

_____

_____

- ☐ Abstract reasoning is more difficult for me.
- → Abstract work includes hypothetical questions, essays, recognizing themes, generalizing ideas to new settings, and flexibility of thinking. Make the abstract more concrete by using visuals and graphic organizer worksheets. Explain to me connections between abstract ideas and everyday concrete situations. Relate the abstract ideas to my areas of interest.
- + I can be excellent at concrete tasks.

- ☐ I miss the big picture because I'm too focused on details.
- → Divide up larger projects into smaller chunks. The smaller chunks can then be put together to create the big picture. For example, a report can be divided into short sections for each chapter. Help me understand things beyond my immediate needs and point of view through volunteering and helping others.
- + I'm good at detailed-orientated tasks such as cataloging books, testing samples in a laboratory, making models, painting, editing, analyzing x-rays, or finding Waldo.

_____

_____

- ☐ I have a good visual memory. I might be good at remembering directions, images, and replaying events or films in my mind. When I have a hard time understanding things, try to make it visual with a diagram, picture, or graphic organizer. When I'm learning something new, remind me to "take a picture of it in my mind." If I'm having difficulty with a writing task that involves creative thinking, ask me if I can first picture it as a movie. ("Can you see the …… in your mind? Can you make the pictures move like in a movie? What happens? What happens next?") I can then draw out the scenes, or write down what happens as I picture it. Remember that some of the visual memories in my mind will be negative ones and can cause me distress years later.
- + A strong visual memory is needed for art, layout, design, movie special effects, camera/ photography.

_____

_____

Educate Others

- ☐ I know that I am different and I might feel like I have come from another planet.
- → Ask me if I feel the same or different from others. Give me a chance to express how I feel. Sometimes a general feeling of being different will be expressed in concrete terms such as "different because I'm not good at sports." Help me make sense of my feelings. "It makes sense you feel different. You're really great at ... but ... is hard for you." Then normalize feeling different by pointing out how other people around me are different too (different skills, physical appearances, challenges, cultural aspects, medical conditions).
- + I can be very accepting of people who are marginalized.

_____

_____

- ☐ I become distressed when things that are important to me do not work out the way I expected.
- → Know that I'm not trying to be difficult, but that it's really challenging for me to see things "working out the wrong way." Communicate that you understand how I feel ("I know this must be really hard for you. It isn't what you expected. You expected ......"). Then give me a sense of hope. ("We can try this again tomorrow.") When appropriate, explain to me why the new result is not wrong. ("The rule is that our client can change her mind on a project whenever she wants.")
- + Trying to do things the right way can make me an excellent employee.

_____

_____

AUTISM RULES

- ☐ I can be a perfectionist.
- → Help me to celebrate my mistakes. "The rule is: The perfect person makes mistakes." Draw a circle and explain that if I try to stay inside the circle and never make mistakes, I won't be able to learn new things or develop inventions. Use examples such as Google that expects failure for new product ideas.
- + I care about my work.

_____

_____

- ☐ I often find other people annoying.
- → The truth is that neurotypicals (those not on the spectrum) are very confusing. They don't say what they're really thinking, they have thousands of rules that are never spoken, their language is full of nonsense sentences ("I smell a rat!"), and they can be critical of those who are different.
- + I can bring a unique perspective to situations.

_____

_____

- ☐ I am easily distracted.
- → Use a planner, routine, structure, written lists, reminders on my phone, and breaks. Help me to organize my work and divide larger assignments into smaller parts. Avoid having me multitask. Learning something with an individual teacher can be easier than in a group situation. I can have a medication consultation for ADD or ADHD if needed.
- + I can be hyper-focused in my area of interest.

Educate Others

_____

_____

- ☐ It's hard for me to accept criticism.
- → Always give criticism when I am calm and out of the situation that is stressing me. Try structuring feedback into my routine. For example, after every project or important event, explore two things that can be improved. Try to start the conversation with a positive statement. Use honesty, logic, and well-thought-out reasoning to explain why you might disagree (see the rule on choosing a social guide in Chapter 3).
- + This is a good reminder of how I am sensitive and that I care about what others think of me.

_____

_____

- ☐ I get depressed.
- → Now that you know my differences, I'm sure you understand why I get depressed living in a world where others don't understand me, and where I don't always understand myself. Help others to understand me by passing on this information and help me to love and accept myself. A medication consultation might be appropriate to help with my depression.
- + I can help others who feel marginalized or depressed by sharing my experiences.

_____

_____

AUTISM RULES

CHAPTER 5

Celebrate Your Differences And If People Don't Like It, Too Bad For Them

Every person I have worked with who is on the spectrum, whether the person's IQ has been in the 9th or the 99th percentile, has shown me a new perspective on life or taught me something new. While there is no one face of autism, people with autism tend to be detail-oriented, visual thinkers, creative, and direct. They tend to care about doing things "the right way." They are people whose greatest strength is to see things differently and who have the courage to make changes in the world.

YOU'RE IN GOOD COMPANY

It's not surprising that when we look at people who are on the spectrum we find that you are in good company. In the following section, we will look at a selection of individuals who are on the spectrum or who have spectrum characteristics, including Michelangelo, Dian Fossey, Sir Anthony Hopkins, Temple Grandin, Dan Aykroyd, Elon Musk, and Greta Thunberg. I hope you will find their lives insightful and encouraging. It is time that we celebrate your differences, and if people don't like it, too bad for them.

MICHELANGELO BUONARROTI SIMONI

*I saw the angel in the marble and I
carved until I set him free.
(Michelangelo on creating the statue of David)*

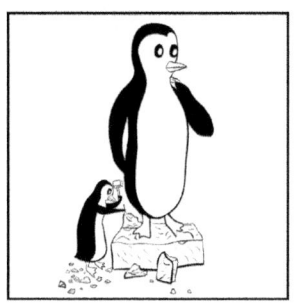

Michelangelo (1475 – 1564) was one of the most talented Italian artists of all time: a painter, sculptor, architect, poet, and engineer whose works include the Sistine Chapel and the David and Pieta statues. Despite his extraordinary talents, his father and uncles did everything they could to discourage his artistic endeavors, including beating him for spending too much time drawing. This only made him more determined to pursue his interests and inspired him to paint one of his first masterpieces of an angel beaten by devils.

In his teens, he became interested in anatomy and studied dissections and visited places like fish markets. He made sketches of the intricate details of both animal and human bones, muscles, veins, and eyes. Michelangelo was always passionate about his art and worked day and night for long hours at a time. He sculpted outdoors regardless of the weather, slept with his clothes and boots on, and took breaks to eat out of necessity more than pleasure.

Michelangelo was an artist who defied conventional society, both in his lack of social interactions and in his original perspectives on art. He continued working until his death at age eighty-eight.

Celebrate Your Differences

DIAN FOSSEY

When you realize the value of all life, you dwell less on what is past and concentrate on the preservation of the future.
(Dian Fossey's final journal entry)

Dian Fossey (1932 – 1985) was a primatologist who spent eighteen years researching and protecting gorillas in Rwanda. Living alone in a hut on the side of a mountain 10,000 feet above sea level, she rejected the textbook approach to gorilla research. Instead of sitting passively and observing, she mimicked the gorilla's movements, sounds, and feeding habits. She munched on wild celery to show submissiveness and made soft purring sounds to express contentment. Her living conditions were rough; she had to overcome poachers, animal traps, torrential rain, mud, revolutions, and the slaughter of gorillas that she had known and loved. In spite of all of this, she slowly gained the trust of the gorillas, and in 1970 she made history when an adult male gorilla she had named "Peanuts" reached out to touch her hand.

Dian's field work saved the lives of countless gorillas by increasing knowledge of their habits, raising funds for protection, and preventing poaching. Dian was murdered in her hut in 1985 and her death still remains a mystery. Her work continues today through the Dian Fossey Gorilla Fund International.

SIR ANTHONY HOPKINS

When I grow up, all I want to be is a little boy.
(Hopkins, 2016)

Sir Anthony Hopkins (Born 1937) is a Welsh actor who has been involved in numerous movies, television shows, and plays including Red Dragon, How the Grinch Stole Christmas, Shadowlands, The Silence of the Lambs, The Elephant Man, All Creatures Great and Small and Hamlet. In The Silence of the Lambs, he played the psychopathic doctor Hannibal Lecter. To prepare for this role he studied interviews of the murderer Charles Manson and discovered a little-known fact– Manson rarely blinked when talking. Anthony incorporated this characteristic into the Hannibal character, giving him an eerie intensity and self-assurance.

Even though he only had 16 minutes of screen time in the whole movie, this detail helped him win an Oscar for his performance. Anthony has also won British Academy film awards and Emmys. In 1993 he was knighted by Queen Elizabeth for his services to the arts.

Anthony's childhood was not as successful. The only child of a baker, he grew up feeling uncomfortable and alone, and had a sense of being unique and outside of the life around him. He remembers that at the age of four he was "totally ill at ease" and had difficulty understanding what others were talking about (Brian Linehan's City Lights, 2015). He describes that he "wasn't too sharp at school," despite his photographic memory. His difficulties with communication and the feeling of not being at ease in the world left him introverted and isolated.

It was Anthony's hunger to communicate with peers that attracted him to the world of acting. As a child he tried to connect with others by using jokes, impersonations, and mimicry. He was talented at performing, and it helped him fit in on the playground, but it also left him feeling uncomfortable, because instead of just being himself, he became a collection of different people. Then, as an adult, he started to perform on stage, but the feeling of not belonging lingered. He didn't feel at home amongst the other actors or in the English National Theatre. It was during this time that he turned to alcohol, perhaps as a way to escape.

After moving to America, his acting became a type of therapy for him. He gained a little something from each part he played, and the characters went into his subconscious where they were processed and integrated. Then, after a particularly bad period of drinking, he realized that his alcohol use was self-destructive, and he stopped drinking and turned to more productive ways of being at ease.

Celebrate Your Differences

Anthony doesn't go to parties or have many friends, but instead focuses on going to work and doing a good job. He learns his scripts meticulously and puts an emphasis on preparation. He visualizes himself doing things he wants to achieve and tells himself that he can do it. He studies people, deconstructs them, pulls their characteristics apart to see what motivates them, and is aware that his view is often different from others.

He was about 70 years old when he was diagnosed with Asperger's. He didn't grow up with the knowledge that the feeling of being different or the struggles to communicate might have been a function of his autism. But I have the sense that he has now found a certain peace with himself and the world around him and that there is truth in the words that he will often say when looking at a picture of himself as a child: "We did okay, kid."

TEMPLE GRANDIN

Using my visualization ability, I observe myself from a distance. I call this my little scientist in the corner, as if I'm a little bird watching my own behavior from up high.
(Grandin, 2006)

There is a professor at Colorado State University who has fans all over the world asking for her autograph and picture. Her fame stretches across the two seemingly separate areas of animal scientist and autism spokesperson. She is smart, compassionate, and exceptionally skilled at what she does.

Temple Grandin (Born 1947) didn't speak until she was three and a half; she had tantrums, showed little interest in other people, and had poor eye contact. She grew up in an era when little was known about autism, and she was misdiagnosed as a child and told that if she could just identify her "psychological injury," she would be cured.

Those around her often failed to understand her and even got in the way of her attempts to meet her own needs. At one point she even built a machine to squeeze her body to calm herself down, but the professionals in her life thought it was too strange and needed to be taken away (Grandin, 2006). Perhaps it was this challenge to be understood that gave her the passion to explain her mind to others and to educate the public on what it's like to go through life with a different perspective.

Temple's perspective involves thinking visually rather than verbally. Her mind is full of video memories and pictures that are ready to use at any moment. Say the word "dessert" to Temple and images will appear in her mind like a Google search. She might see recently-consumed cake pops and chocolate cake, strawberry shortcake, and coffee ice cream she ate as a child (Cooper-White, 2014). Her memories are usually grouped together based on association, with one subject skipping to another if there is some type of connection between them. As she explains in her autobiography, "Thought does not have to be verbal or sequential to be real" (Grandin, 2006).

It is Temple's visualization skill that has made her successful in her career as an animal scientist. She is particularly famous for designing facilities to handle cattle and hogs. She can scan through her video-like memories of items she has worked on and put the pieces together in unique ways, visualizing animals going through her design before it's built, viewing it from different angles, and finding potential problems.

When she is asked to examine facilities where animals are scared, she has an excellent attention to detail that helps her identify the problems – a spot of sunlight, an unexpected shadow, a plastic water bottle on the ground. Her work to reduce animal suffering has resulted in numerous awards. She was named one of Time Magazine's most 100 influential people in the world, and was also listed as one of the top 10 college professors in the country by Ceoworld Magazine.

Temple is keen to pass on her knowledge and does it through teaching, interviews, books, DVDs, conferences, and a movie about her life (Jackson, 2010). She gives out her personal phone number to students and tells them to call her whenever they have a question. As for retirement she says, "I probably won't stop until I'm incapacitated" (Phifer, 2018).

DAN AYKROYD

I feel like an alien.
(Aykroyd, 2018)

Dan Aykroyd was born in Canada in 1952 and was diagnosed with autism after his wife persuaded him to see a doctor. Known for being a musician, comedian, actor, and businessman, Dan has starred in several shows and movies including Saturday Night Live, The Blues Brothers, Ghostbusters, Dragnet, Driving Miss Daisy, and My Girl. Dan's family of origin has a long history of fascination with the supernatural. His great-grandfather was a mystic, and his father was raised in a home that had frequent séances and spiritualist activities. Dan describes how he eagerly read his grandfather's diaries on spiritualism and joined a society which studies the paranormal. It is this obsession with interacting with the dead and the afterworld that led him to write the script for Ghostbusters. As he points out, paranormal events such as a trumpet floating around the room with voices coming out can be very entertaining.

ELON MUSK

I reinvented electric cars and I'm sending people to Mars on a rocket ship — did you think I was also going to be a chill, normal dude?
(Musk, 2021)

Elon Musk (Born 1971) is a soft-spoken, gifted engineer who grew up in South Africa. He believed he was "insane" as a child because his mind was "exploding with ideas," so it is not surprising that he has enterprises in a variety of fields including electric vehicles, energy, and the quest for humanity to become a multi-planet species. He is the co-founder and leader of Tesla, SpaceX, Neuralink, and The Boring Company. He is the owner of Twitter.

Elon spent most of his childhood reading books and building rockets by himself. When his parents divorced around the age of 10, he went to live with his father, Errol. Elon had felt sorry for him living alone and had thought that he could be a good companion. This early decision turned out to be a huge mistake. Errol has been reported as being significantly mentally and physically abusive, and Elon describes him as a "terrible human being" who "can take any situation no matter how good it is and make it bad." According to Elon, his father has committed almost every crime you can think of.

Unfortunately, Elon's school environment paralleled his miserable experience at home. His younger age, smaller size, and interest in books made him a target for school bullies. On one occasion he was kicked in the head, thrown down a flight of stairs, and had his head bashed against the ground. The injury was so bad that he had to be hospitalized. For many of my clients on the spectrum, childhood trauma often occurs in the context of greater social isolation, which makes it so much harder for the person to be heard and helped.

It was perhaps due to the brutality of his world that he began to create other more hospitable realities. He developed a computer game at age 12 that involved defeating an alien spaceship, and he became a master in Dungeons and Dragons. At age 17 Elon escaped to Canada to begin his studies, and from there he moved to the United States.

Elon's first business, Zip2, was created with his brother, Kimbal. Their idea was revolutionary for the times —an online directory with maps. They rented a small office in Palo Alto where they lived and worked seven days a week, sleeping on the couch or beanbag chair and showering at the YMCA. However, when Elon made millions from the sale of the company, he didn't retire to a glamorous lifestyle like many others would have done. Instead, he invested most of the profits into his next business, one of the world's first online banks, PayPal.

This early pattern of drive and hard work can be seen in his current enterprises. Over the years, he has slept on factory floors because he didn't have time to go home and shower, and he has worked throughout departments such as general assembly, the body shop, and the paint shop. He rarely takes vacations, and in one period of 12 years he only took two weeks off. He has worked so hard that he says that his "brain and heart hurt."

Celebrate Your Differences

For Elon though, it is not about the money but the significance of what he is doing. When he started SpaceX, he didn't expect it to succeed, but he put 100 million dollars of his own money into the company. He felt passionate about the possibility of ordinary people going into space, and he needed to own the company to have the freedom to do the engineering the way he wanted. In 2008 the SpaceX rocket had its third consecutive failure, Tesla was almost bankrupt, and he was going through a divorce, but his desire to keep trying was so strong that he states that he would have only given up if he was "dead or completely incapacitated."

Elon talks about having once felt that his companies were like the scrappy little kid fighting the great sumo wrestlers. Some of those wrestlers are short sellers who bet on his company stocks going down and do everything they can to present them in a negative light. Others are his personal heroes such as Neil Armstrong and Gene Cernan who questioned the safety and quality of his spaceflight work and testified in Congress against his enterprises. Not only does this make Elon's objectives harder to achieve, but their attacks are emotionally painful for him, something he describes as "hurtful."

It's possible that Elon felt the same in his childhood when he faced his classmates or his father. They were the people in his life who should have been there to help, not hurt. Perhaps if Elon's father and peers had taken the time to have a clearer vision of him, if they had understood his autism, they could have seen him for who he is — an intelligent and creative individual whose strengths and challenges happen to be very different from others.

GRETA THUNBERG

Given the right circumstances — being different is a superpower.
(Thunberg, 2020)

Greta (Born 2003) is an environmental activist from Sweden. She was diagnosed with autism following a period of severe depression where she stopped eating, laughing, and talking. Her parents discovered that she had been bullied at school, pushed down on the playground, and shunned for her differences. Then one day she watched a film in school about how much garbage there was in the ocean, and she began to read about carbon emissions and environmental damage. She suddenly saw how people's choices such as flying or shopping had a cost to the environment, and she found it hard to understand the lack of response from leaders. In an attempt to make a difference, she skipped school one Friday and stood alone outside the Swedish Parliament with a sign that read "School Strike for Climate." She posted her picture to her twenty followers on Instagram, and she quickly attracted the interest of organizations, newspapers, and other young people.

Greta went on to give high-profile speeches, meet with world leaders, and sail across the Atlantic for a UN climate action summit. Within a year, her movement had grown to millions of students across the globe walking out of school to protest. However, not all the attention that Greta has attracted has been positive. There are those who don't believe in climate change or in supporting a youth who seems to hold so much power. Others have difficulty with her direct style of speaking and her refusal to back down from her ideals. But this has not stopped her from continuing to speak out for her cause, and she has won numerous awards, including Time magazine's Person of the Year and nominations for the Nobel Peace Prize.

YOU CAN LEARN FROM SUCCESS

In this next section we will look in greater depth at the lives of three people diagnosed with autism or with autism characteristics — Susan Boyle, Albert Einstein, and Satoshi Tajiri. By studying their stories, you can learn from their experiences and understand the specific strategies they used to thrive. Questions from their stories that I want to answer are: How are they different from most neurotypicals? What were their struggles? And what were the factors that helped them to succeed? The strategies that helped them to succeed will be listed as rules that you can apply to your own life as needed.

Celebrate Your Differences

SUSAN BOYLE

*If you have a dream, it's never too late
to give it your best shot.*
(Boyle, 2014)

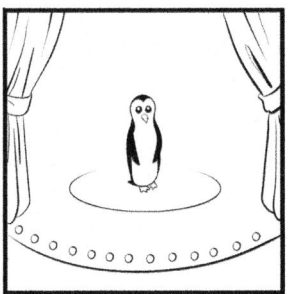

In 2009 a middle aged, unemployed woman stepped onto the stage of Britain's Got Talent. The judges asked her a question about where she lived, and she struggled to answer. She then tried to make some jokes, and the audience cringed at her offbeat humor. The judge, Simon Cowell, rolled his eyes with the exasperated look of someone who didn't want a contestant to waste his precious time.

When she shared that she was trying to be a professional singer, the audience started laughing at how ridiculous that was. One thing was clear. She had been on the stage for less than sixty seconds and most of the people in the room had turned against her. The judges then asked her why she hadn't already succeeded, and she replied, "I haven't been given the chance before." For her audition she chose the song, "I Dreamed a Dream" from Les Miserables. The original song, written in French, was titled "I had dreamed of another life."

Up to this point, Susan Boyle's life had been a challenging one. She was born in 1961 in a small town in Blackburn, Scotland, the youngest of nine children. Her parents were told that because she had suffered a lack of oxygen at birth "she would never be anything" and that they shouldn't expect too much of her.

She screamed a lot, had difficulty sleeping at night, and would only sleep during the day if her dad was wearing his red sweater. Frequent hospital visits led to a diagnosis of "hyperactive" and her family lived in fear that she would be put in an institution one day like her Uncle Michael.

Some of Susan's earliest memories are of feeling that she did not fit in like other people, of knowing that she was different. She remembers standing alone on the playground struggling to understand social rules and being confused as to why others weren't her friend. She knew that she wanted to please her peers, but when she tried to entertain them by acting out television characters, they laughed at her. When she was excited, she was told she was too loud. When she was sad or angry, she was told she was too emotional. Susan always had words in her head, things she wanted to say, but her thoughts got stuck as if trapped behind an invisible barrier. At other times she was just told that she sounded too adult.

A friend of Susan's who was at school with her said that Susan was usually on her own watching others, and when she did interact, people made fun of her because she was not the same as everyone else (NorKalCay, 2013). They called her names and didn't allow her to play with them. Her lack of social interaction made the gap between herself and her peers grow larger, and by the time she reached middle school, she was withdrawn, isolated, and bullied. On one occasion, children followed her home from school, pushed her into a ditch, and stubbed out a cigarette on her jacket.

The first time Susan sang solo was during a Burns Day competition at elementary school. She was ten years old and afraid that her singing would end the way things normally did, with everyone making fun of her. The only reason she even tried was that she didn't want to disappoint her music teacher. But when she finished singing, Susan noticed something very different. People were smiling, someone in the audience said "Well done," and her classmates clapped.

Where the playground social interactions had failed, singing succeeded. For the first time in her life, Susan had found a way to connect with others and to know what it felt like to be actually good at something, to make people around her happy. As Susan describes in her autobiography, "When you've been jeered at, told to shut up, sit still, stop being silly, there's a cacophony of noise constantly rolling around inside your head. When I was singing, it was peaceful" (Boyle, 2010, p 65).

Susan's ability to sing her way out of social isolation can be seen in early videos of her as a young adult in pubs and social gatherings. While everyone else is talking and laughing together, Susan is alone. There's no group of people wishing her luck or walking onto the stage with her. But when she starts to sing, she looks at the crowd and they look back at her, she makes eye contact, she smiles, she stares directly into the camera, and the chattering in the room turns to an attentive silence. There is the sense that in this moment she knows that she is valued.

Susan has shared that she has high anxiety from feelings of inferiority and her struggle to be accepted by others (NorCalKay, 2016). Singing helps Susan to chase these challenges away. As she got older, she sang whenever she could. She sang at the Happy Valley Pub, social clubs, and village events. She auditioned for Opportunity Knocks and other talent shows. She sang through periods of unemployment and the grief of her mother's death. It was an escape from the stresses of life.

When Susan walked onto the stage of Britain's Got Talent she had already experienced a lifetime of rejection. She was the girl who had been told she had brain damage and wouldn't amount to much. She was the one that the Britain's Got Talent audience laughed at and the judges underestimated. But within a few seconds of Susan's singing, the beauty and strength of her voice melted away their cynicism. As one judge noted, it was the biggest surprise they had seen on the show in three years, and nobody was laughing at her now.

Within a week, 100 million people had watched her audition on YouTube. There were journalists, photographers, interviews, phone calls, and requests for autographs. Becoming a celebrity overnight can be challenging for anyone, but it was especially hard for Susan. Journalists harassed her hoping to get a reaction, and she responded with anger, yelling, and tears. She had to listen to people calling her arrogant, insecure, spoiled, fake, and moody (Jordan, 2009). By the time the final show came, she was exhausted and under so much pressure that she saw her second place as a failure, and she checked into an inpatient clinic.

Before she became a celebrity, she had spent her days at home with her cat, Pebbles, or walking up and down the rows of shops on her high street. But now that she was famous, her days were filled with changing locations and unfamiliar faces. She had to communicate with managers and fans and try to meet their high expectations. Journalists watched and photographed her every action then published it in disparaging articles. Others made fun of her humor or the way she looked. It was as though Susan was back at school being chased by the bullies, only now she couldn't run home to her family. She couldn't take solace in the familiar. Some journalists have talked about Susan's "hooded look" where she puts her head down, stops talking, and withdraws, leaving those around her confused. Did someone do something she didn't like? Was the restaurant menu taken away too quickly? Susan says that during these moments she experiences panic, anxiety, and the "terror of life" (Johnston, 2014).

Trying to make sense of all of her unusual reactions, Susan came to two conclusions, one was that the brain damage label didn't fit her; the other was that she didn't experience life like everyone else. It was three years after her rise to fame that Susan finally found the answer. She was on the autism spectrum.

When she received the diagnosis, she felt a great relief. There was a name for what she had, a way forward where others could finally understand and support her. "I think people will treat me better because they will have a much greater understanding of who I am and why I do the things I do," she explains (Deveney, 2013).

That's not to say that Susan doesn't still struggle with communicating or that she doesn't become frustrated or withdrawn. She does. But now she and her team know that simple strategies like taking a break and walking away will help her. They also know she will always be back.

We will now take a look at the rules that helped her succeed and that can be applied to your own life.

Celebrate Your Differences

SUCCESS STRATEGY:
USE A LANGUAGE THAT WORKS FOR YOU

Susan wanted to communicate with other people, but words didn't work for her. People misread her intentions, intelligence, and emotions. They became angry, made fun of her, and laughed. It is understandable that in this world of words, Susan was left feeling anxious, judged, and insecure. But the young girl who discovered that people smiled when she sang is the same one who feels peaceful on the stage today. It is here that she connects with others, feels appreciated, and expresses emotions that can't be put into words. The same is true when she's in the recording studio. For Susan, singing creates a bubble of safety between her and the clutter of life. In her autobiography she describes it this way:

"I feel that I have come home to a place where I know I am safe. I become a calm person, a person who knows her value, a person who has been given the great privilege of doing that she does best without any distractions. My only conversation is with the song" (Boyle, 2010). Using a language that works for her has resulted in the sale of more than 25 million records, numerous awards, worldwide tours, charity performances, and performances for Pope Benedict XVI, President Obama, and the Queen of England.

Examples of different languages that might work for you include painting, animation, comic book design, music, poetry, song writing, pottery, creative writing, culinary arts, and creation and use of memes.

SUCCESS STRATEGY:
FIND PEOPLE WHO BELIEVE IN YOU

Susan had plenty of people in her life who put her down, but she also found people to lift her up. It was Susan's mother, Bridget, who first said that she should audition for Britain's Got Talent, telling her that she thought she could win. Bridget died two years before the audition, and Susan entered the show partly as a tribute to her, knowing that she would be proud of her efforts and feeling as if her mother was with her spiritually. "There has been some type of intervention," Susan said, "She has had a word with someone upstairs, because I wouldn't have had this otherwise" (Deveney, 2013). Susan also found a singing coach, Fred O'Neil, who taught her for years and supported her. She felt that these people were walking onto the stage with her to help her face an audience that would expect failure. Susan has shared that all she needed was someone to believe in her, someone to say that she can do it.

SUCCESS STRATEGY: FAIL FAST, FAIL OFTEN

Susan has a long history of failure. She didn't win her school singing competition at age ten. She wasn't selected for the TV shows Opportunity Knocks and My Kind of People. Singing in karaoke nights and the Happy Valley Pub never made her famous, and neither did singing at church. In fact, she didn't even win Britain's Got Talent. Susan failed fast, usually not even getting a callback, and she failed often.

It's clear that Susan didn't wait around for years trying to perfect her craft before putting it out there. Instead, she invited failure in by entering events that could help her reach her goal of becoming a professional singer. The lack of success was frustrating and disappointing, but from each failure Susan gained an essential new skill and received a piece of feedback or information that helped her move forward.

At the school competition she learned that she was good at something and could make people happy, at the pub she began to connect with the audience and became encouraged to sing in other places, at the audition for Opportunity Knocks she developed a determination to do better, and at My Kind of People she found a teacher who helped her enter Britain's Got Talent - where she lost and became a professional singer.

Celebrate Your Differences

ALBERT EINSTEIN

I very rarely think in words at all. A thought comes, and I may try to express it in words afterwards.
(Einstein, 1916)

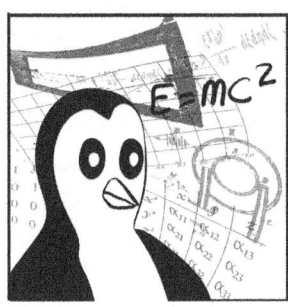

Nobody personifies the image of genius more than the wild-haired, disheveled, Albert Einstein. His intelligence was admired so much that after his death someone stole his brain to find out what made him so different. They cut it into 240 pieces, put the pieces in jars, stored them in a box under a beer cooler, and sent them around the world to be investigated.

Einstein never asked for this, he had wanted to be cremated and to have his ashes secretly scattered. But when you come up with the Theory of Relativity, the formula $E=mc^2$, win a Nobel Prize in physics, and are asked to be the president of Israel, people begin to wonder how you got there.

Albert Einstein was born in Germany on March 14, 1879. He was a quiet child, who played by himself with puzzles, blocks, and houses of cards that reached fourteen stories high. His speech was delayed, and at one point his family was afraid that he might never communicate. When he finally began to talk, he had a habit of repeating sentences by mouthing them to himself. He was easily frustrated and prone to tantrums. He struck his music teacher with a chair, threw a large bowling ball at his younger sister, and knocked a hole in his sister's head with a child's hoe.

Einstein said that he felt separated from other people, as if there was a pane of glass between himself and others. He viewed himself as "somewhat odd, uncommunicative, and solitary." His self-described "obstinate sense of detachment" and need for solitude increased as he aged. His assistant Leopold Infeld thought that Einstein could understand others when it came to logical matters but struggled to grasp emotional issues and feelings that weren't related to his own life.

Academically, Einstein ignored the subjects that bored him. He disliked French and Greek, and would later describe himself as having a poor memory for words. In class, his peers answered questions quickly, but Einstein often hesitated, and when he got answers wrong, teachers inflicted him with whacks on the knuckles. At one point the Greek teacher told him that he would never amount to anything, that he was wasting everyone's time, and that he should immediately leave the school. But Einstein embraced the subjects that interested him, excelling in math and science. Around the age of five, his father showed him a compass to distract him from an illness that he was recovering from. This was a key moment in awakening Einstein's scientific curiosity. He became immediately intrigued by the needle's ability to point north no matter how he turned it, and this made him think about the hidden forces behind material things. By the age of thirteen, he had independently studied his school's entire math curriculum, proving almost all of the theories for himself, and finding original approaches to problems.

Einstein felt that his natural curiosity developed more when he had the freedom to choose what he wanted to study. When a subject bored him, he would skip classes and lectures. However, this independent spirit caused professors to dislike him and made it difficult for him to obtain recommendations for work. He spoke his mind, questioned authority, and did things his own way rather than following instructions. At one point, his failure to listen caused him to explode his lab experiment and injure his right hand.

After college, he sent out numerous letters for assistant positions but was the only student in his graduating class who failed to get placed. Discouraged, he tried private tutoring but struggled with this too. In one tutoring position, he was fired because he refused to sit at the dinner table, as he found the family's conversation too dull. It took Einstein two years to find regular employment as a low-level patent inspector.

Celebrate Your Differences

Even though Einstein had difficulties getting along with others, there is plenty of evidence that he enjoyed being with people, especially in situations that concerned his areas of interest. In college, he formed close friendships with students who were studying science, and he met with them regularly to discuss theories and share class notes. He could also be very playful and had a wonderful rapport with children. He took the time to personally answer many of their letters, describing scientific concepts, encouraging, and explaining everything from the necessity of sunlight to the importance of collaboration.

For Einstein, embracing his interests was a way of being, a center that he would consistently come back to no matter what he was doing. It wasn't so much a matter of choice but a reflection of how his mind worked. We see this in his letters to his first wife Mileva Maric where he would drift back and forth between romantic talk and scientific discussion. The same pattern appears in his autobiography, or "obituary" as he calls it, where he starts by sharing a few details about his life and then drifts into geometry. He catches this drift, noting that he has allowed his thoughts to interrupt his barely started obituary. A page later he writes, "And now back to the obituary," and he gives just a few more life details before returning to the science again. He stops himself again saying, "Is this supposed to be an obituary?" He then writes that the most important thing about him is how he thinks, as if giving himself permission to do what he likes best –share his scientific ideas.

Here are some of the strategies that helped him succeed and that can be applied to your own life:

SUCCESS STRATEGY: PASSIONATELY EMBRACE YOUR INTERESTS

All the postmortem investigations of Einstein's brain gave no clear answers as to what made him a genius or helped him to succeed. It is not in the weight of his cortex or in the density of his neurons that we find the answer but in his own understanding of his mind. When asked about his success, Einstein often said that it was due to his passionate curiosity. Young Einstein didn't just build a fourteen-story house of cards on his first try. He persevered and improved regardless of how many times the cards collapsed. Building the perfect house required taking what he learned from each failure and trying again and again, knowing that some of his ideas would lead to nowhere. Einstein described himself as being stubborn. I would call him passionate and committed to his areas of interest.

SUCCESS STRATEGY:
BE AN INDEPENDENT THINKER

An explosion in a lab, unemployment, low grades from poor attendance, and lack of support from teachers were all symptoms of Einstein's independent thinking, but it was ultimately this independence that allowed him to thrive. His theories required rejecting many of the accepted notions of his day. How could he have done that if he had stuck to conventional wisdom?

SUCCESS STRATEGY:
ASK FOR SUPPORT FROM FAMILY AND FRIENDS

Einstein's family encouraged his interests and helped him to develop his talents. His Uncle Jakob Einstein was an engineer with skills in algebra. He noticed Einstein's love of math and gave him challenging theories to solve that went far beyond his elementary school level. Einstein enjoyed solving the problems and often came back for more. Another uncle Caesar Koch gave him a steam-driven engine that helped him to first notice the connections between heat and force.

Einstein also had practical support. His friend Marcel Grossman was especially helpful. He would often lend his notebook to Einstein so that he could study for exams and he helped him out of his discouraging two-year period of unemployment by finding him a job in the Swiss Patent Office. Einstein was so thankful for Grossman's support that he dedicated his doctoral thesis to him.

Others gave Einstein help in his day-to-day life. This included reminding him to eat, telling him to change his clothes, recovering belongings that he had left somewhere, and opening the door when he didn't have his house keys. He once forgot his suitcase at a host's house, and the host said to his parents, "That man will never amount to anything because he can't remember anything." Fortunately, there were people in his life who could help him with details that he probably thought of as insignificant.

SUCCESS STRATEGY: CONSIDER EMPLOYMENT WITH ROUTINE, SECURITY, AND FEW SOCIAL DEMANDS

1905 is known as Einstein's golden year. It was this year that he developed his Theory of Relativity, the formula E=mc2, and published several papers that transformed physics. It is interesting that this was also the year when he had what he called his "cobblers trade" position at the patent office. The employment was well-paid and had a structured eight-hour work day. The work was easy for him, and unlike his university studies that had been too focused on the past, this position focused on the future by reviewing plans for new inventions. This kept his mind alert and in his areas of interest, without being so stressful that it took away from his own creative abilities. He had a director who was logical and consistent and who appreciated Einstein's qualities, even giving him a raise a few months after being hired. It is not surprising that Einstein referred to it as, "that worldly cloister where I hatched my most beautiful ideas."

SATOSHI TAJIRI

*When people who want to make games gather,
there's a chance a game will be born.*
(Tajiri, 2004)

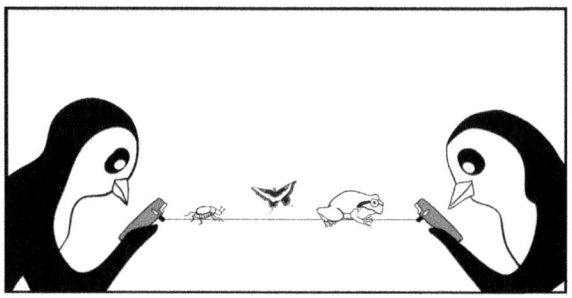

Few games have captured the imagination of both children and adults like Pokemon, the pocket monsters that can be collected, raised, battled, and traded. They have become an international multi-media phenomenon with games, cards, anime, films, comics, books, merchandise, tournaments, festivals, and more. The creator of this billion-dollar franchise is an autistic man, Satoshi Tajiri.

Satoshi was born in 1965 and grew up just outside of Tokyo in an area with rivers, rice fields, and forests. A favorite activity for children in the area was to find beetles by smearing honey on trees. Tajiri became fascinated with the insects and spent hours investigating their habits. His family didn't have honey to use for traps, but when he discovered that beetles liked to sleep under stones during the day, he placed large rocks around the trees to attract them.

His quest for insects expanded to rivers, where he scooped up crayfish and searched in air bubbles and under sticks. He found frogs and tadpoles with translucent bellies that looked odd and exciting. He liked the way the different insects moved, and he brought various specimen home to study. The more he searched, the more he found, making him the best insect hunter amongst his peers and earning himself the nickname "Dr. Bug."

Celebrate Your Differences

As his town became more urban, the bugs started to disappear, and his interests shifted to video games. His new obsession quickly took over his life, and he began to ignore his school work and sneak off to various arcades during the day. He especially enjoyed playing Space Invaders, and he thought about how he could make a sequel. In his final year of high school when his peers were applying to college, Satoshi didn't even have enough credits to graduate. At the time, video games were new in Japan, and his parents thought of him as a delinquent who was as bad as a shoplifter. Satoshi became an outcast leading a double life, but he eventually managed to complete enough make-up classes to finish school, and his father found him employment at the Tokyo Electric Power Company. Satoshi turned it down.

Instead of working at the company, he spent his days in video arcades becoming more and more fascinated with the intricate details of the games, even taking apart a Nintendo system to see how it operated. He wanted to know how he could play the games faster and more successfully. There were plenty of rumors in the arcades about secret features in the games. For example, if you played a certain way, a phantom plane or a red dog was supposed to appear. Most of these rumors turned out to be false, and he realized that it was hard to find good information.

Wanting to correct this, Satoshi started his own publication, Game Freak. He knew it wouldn't be a glamorous publication, but he thought that if he could provide accurate details about strategies, reviews, and rumors, then gamers would buy it. He started with just a few handwritten pages that he photocopied and stapled together, and he took them to a store that was willing to put five copies on its shelf. Two very interesting things happened with his magazine. The first was that it quickly became so popular that Satoshi began to have it professionally printed. The second was that he started to be contacted by other like-minded people who were skilled video game players and who had tips to share about games. Satoshi and his new friends began to meet as a group to talk about the games, and they talked about the possibility of making their own. One of these gamers was Ken Sugimori, the man who would eventually illustrate the original 151 Pokemon characters.

If you ask Satoshi what inspired him to make the first Pokemon games, he will tell you about the communication cable. In the 1980s, Nintendo produced a handheld console called "Game Boy" that allowed gamers to play outside of the home. It came with a cable for players to connect with each other while competing. But when Satoshi saw this cable he saw something very different—the possibility of exchange. He imagined living organisms moving back and forth across the cable. It would be a whole new way to interact. Not competitive, but collaborative, where the "I want that" could become a reality with one person passing something to another.

Satoshi had forgotten all about his bug collecting, but suddenly this childhood obsession merged with his adult interests. He remembered how he had searched for interesting insects to examine, raise, and hold, and he thought about children in more urban areas who couldn't have the experiences he had enjoyed when younger. He knew how much fun it was to be the best hunter and to find different types of species. Then Satoshi began to ask himself an interesting question — What if children could collect similar creatures in a video game?

Satoshi and his team started to design creatures that could go through metamorphosis and that could only be caught in specific ways. There were monsters that looked like butterflies, frogs, crabs, caterpillars, and more. Satoshi had especially loved the tadpoles and frogs of his childhood with their translucent bellies and visible circular intestines, and he transformed them into his favorite character, Poliwag, a blue creature with a swirl on its stomach.

Despite the international success of Pokemon, Satoshi has remained relatively unknown. This is unusual in the gaming world where designers often embrace their fame. He doesn't do many interviews or appearances, and he is described by others as being reclusive and eccentric. He keeps unusual work hours, sleeping for twelve hours and then working for twenty-four, and he says that it is often during the night that he will come up with his best ideas.

In one of his rare interviews, Satoshi explained that he wanted to "go against the grain" as a designer. Going against the grain meant living life differently. Satoshi didn't stand next to trees smearing on honey and waiting for bugs but went out alone and searched in unusual places. He wasn't connecting with his

Celebrate Your Differences

peers in class but was on his bike looking for secret video arcades. He couldn't talk to his parents about his passions, and his teachers must have thought of him as oppositional and disobedient. Going against the grain meant living on the margins of society. This must have been especially hard in the Japanese culture where inclusion is highly valued.

In the Pokemon anime there is a character called "Ash" who Satoshi says is himself as a child. Ash spends most of his childhood playing alone, but he greatly values friendships and being with others. He sees friends as people to play with and talk to, and he wants his Pokemon team to feel like one big family. The anime has messages about sticking together, protecting one another, bringing in new family members, and making them feel welcome.

When talking about the Pokemon game, Satoshi says that his goal was to foster these kinds of sentiments in the players. He wanted to make a game that involved interactive communication, where people could play in the same space. It would be one-on-one, with structure, respect, and rules. A place where people like himself could make friends. In developing this new space where he could play and communicate, Satoshi gave a gift of friendship to others. It is not surprising that one of the best known Pokemon slogans is, "Get out and play together."

Here are some of the strategies that helped Satoshi succeed and that can be applied to your own life:

SUCCESS STRATEGY: START WHERE YOU CAN

When Satoshi began putting his skills into the world, he didn't wait until he had the means to produce a perfect product that was well packaged and marketed. Instead, he started where he could with a simple handwritten, stapled-together magazine of five copies. It was this humble beginning that grew into a community, a company, and ultimately his video game production. Satoshi had the courage to start small, where he could, with what he had.

SUCCESS STRATEGY: DEVELOP A COMMUNITY

When Satoshi first started playing video games, he was an outcast, a Japanese youth who was marginalized. There were no video game clubs at his school, and his parents were afraid he would end up unemployed. But when Satoshi started Game Freak magazine, he formed a bridge between himself and others who were also interested in gaming. They met, they talked, they shared ideas and had deeper conversations about the things they were interested in. There was nobody to tell them they had talked too long about one subject, and they weren't negatively judged for their passion. It was a safe place to learn, explore new ideas, and find validation. His magazine community grew into a company that asked every employee to design their own Pokemon. They voted on which ones they thought were best and worked on them together. Satoshi's creativity flourished when embedded in community.

SUCCESS STRATEGY: FIND MENTORS

Satoshi had mentors who had a profound effect on his success by opening doors to his career, increasing his confidence, and teaching him new skills. When talking about his mentors, Satoshi says that he had memorized every piece of their advice.

Satoshi appreciated it when a mentor was open-minded and gave him the freedom to do as he pleased, within the constraints of some basic direction. For example, one mentor asked Satoshi, "Wouldn't it be better if the receiver moved?" but left it up to Satoshi to figure out how this would happen in the context of the game. He didn't demand it, but merely suggested it. Satoshi describes this type of guidance as 'hints' that helped him turn his small ideas into explosive ones.

Celebrate Your Differences

SUCCESS STRATEGY: USE YOUR DETERMINATION

Satoshi had always thought that Nintendo would reject the first Pokemon game because the concept would be too difficult for them to grasp, but this didn't make him walk away from the project. He chose to develop it anyway, and he worked hard on it for several years. He invested so much time and money that several of his employees left Game Freak. When he finally took the finished game to Nintendo, he said he felt like a baseball player sliding into second base, even though he knew he was going to be out.

This determination was evident early in Satoshi's life. He once spent six months looking for a legendary arcade that was rumored to be cheaper than others in his region. He searched around the neighborhoods and asked everyone who was spreading the rumor. Then, when he found it, he rode his bicycle there instead of taking the train so that he could save his money for playing the games.

When Satoshi talks about what he has done to get where he is, he gives the impression that his hard work is normal. He sees a problem, finds a solution, and takes the necessary steps. In the interview where he is talking about creating the first copies of his Game Freak magazine, he describes how he wanted a Dig Dug character on the cover but was doing the magazine by himself and found drawing difficult. To resolve this, he stared at the Dig Dug on the arcade game screen and figured out how the dots were laid out and then drew it one dot at a time.

It is easy to see the similarities with his Pokemon character Ash who is often telling his team to "give it a try" and that he "won't give up." "If I give up," he says, "It'll all be over."

YOU CAN LEARN FROM FICTIONAL CHARACTERS

*I wish people understood that human
interaction exhausts me.*

When you feel different from those around you, it can be validating to discover someone similar to yourself on television or in a novel. It can broaden your perspective and open up discussions about strengths and challenges. Below I have listed some of my favorite fictional characters with autism characteristics that I have come to know and love. As more people with autism are represented in the arts, my hope is that we will see a greater diversity of all types of people on the spectrum.

JULIA

*Play, play, play!
(Julia)*

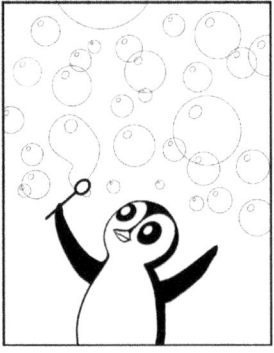

Julia is a four-year-old who moves to Sesame Street and becomes friends with Elmo. In this TV series she likes to play, chase, sing, paint, blow bubbles, and spend time with her toy bunny Fluffster. She doesn't like finger painting or loud noises. When Big Bird meets Julia, he worries that she might not like him because she doesn't respond, but Alan explains that she wants people to know that she has autism and that she often does things differently. She jumps when playing tag and needs to be asked to do things more than once. The other characters on Sesame Street note that she does things "in a Julia kind of way."

The show includes some scenes of Julia taking breaks and doing deep breathing to calm down, and it explores ideas such as finding common ground and respecting differences. We also learn about several of Julia's strengths including playing I-spy and finding patterns (Sesame Street, 2018).

Julia, Elmo, and Alan also answer viewers' questions about how to be a good friend to someone with autism. This includes understanding schedules, differences in eating habits, communicating with pictures, and play (Today, 2018).

CHRISTOPHER BOONE

I like looking up at the sky in the garden at night.... that makes you seem very small, and if you have difficult things in your life, it is nice to think that they are what is called negligible...
(Boone)

We find Christopher Boone in Mark Haddon's novel, 'The Curious Incident of the Dog in the Night-Time.' When fifteen-year-old Christopher finds a murdered dog in his neighbor's yard, he decides to investigate. Using his keen sense of observation, logic, and a courage to keep going even when it's difficult, he not only solves the mystery of the dog but also discovers some family secrets that change his life.

Christopher's character is beautifully written and easy to empathize with. The first-person narrative takes us into his thoughts, feelings, and questions about the world around him. We learn about his love of math and science, his need for maps and order, and how he likes to make diagrams of his choices in his head.

His interests are woven into the story through scientific discussions on a variety of topics such as why the night sky is dark, what elements go into a formula for fear, and how the population of frogs in a pond can vary. The book also reveals many of Christopher's challenges. He hates to be touched, he believes that seeing four yellow cars in a row will make it a bad day, he can become very anxious when things do not go as expected, and he finds people difficult to understand because they "do a lot of talking without using any words."

Although Christopher is just one autistic person, he reminds me of so many of the people I have worked with. This is an innovative and moving novel that is hard to put down.

DR. SHAUN MURPHY

I just did a test. Every toilet paper roll in this restroom has the paper hanging over, not under, and they were installed by professionals.
(Dr. Murphy)

In this TV series, 'The Good Doctor,' Dr. Shaun Murphy is hired by a prestigious hospital. His mentor, Dr. Glassman, believes in his abilities to be a surgeon and puts his own position as hospital president on the line by supporting him. However, other people question Dr. Murphy's skills. How can he be a surgeon when he struggles to communicate? Will his autism be a liability? Can he support his team when needed?

We see Shaun struggling with many of the issues that other autistic people face, such as trying to learn the rules of the neurotypical world while staying true to his own values and needs. We also learn that Shaun has experienced a difficult past of homelessness and the death of his brother. These issues are set against the backdrop of all the usual drama of a hospital show.

'The Good Doctor' is produced by David Shore, the creator of House, so he brings his years of experience in writing about a brilliant doctor who challenges social norms. Shaun is played by actor Freddie Highmore, who appears to be sensitive to the fact that Shaun is just one person and is not supposed to represent everyone on the autism spectrum (Access, 2017).

We learn how Shaun's thinking differs from others with his excellent visual memory, difficulties processing sensory information, and his need for routine. The only piece that doesn't seem quite right is how Freddie portrays Shaun's lack of eye contact. At times it can appear slightly off beat, but perhaps this is more of an example of how hard it can be to learn a new pattern of eye contact, whether you are on the spectrum or not.

Overall, The Good Doctor is one of my favorite shows.

SAM GARDNER

The campus is on a hill, and I don't like the idea of living at an angle.
(Gardner)

'Atypical' is a coming-of-age story on Netflix, staring Sam Gardner, an eighteen-year-old teenager who loves penguins, Antarctica, and drawing. Diagnosed with autism at the age of four, we meet him in his final year of high school where he's attempting to become more independent and start dating. Keir Gilchrist is outstanding in this role and plays it with incredible consistency, often giving the viewer the perspective of what it is like to have a mind that works differently or how it is to be overwhelmed by sensory information.

Season Two includes autistic actors who are members of a support group that Sam attends. The story also focuses on Sam's parents and his sister, and we learn about their own secrets and struggles, sending the message that we are all in our own ways trying to find our place in the world.

The show has sexual content, bad language, alcohol, drugs, and some violence.

SEEING THINGS DIFFERENTLY IS YOUR GREATEST STRENGTH

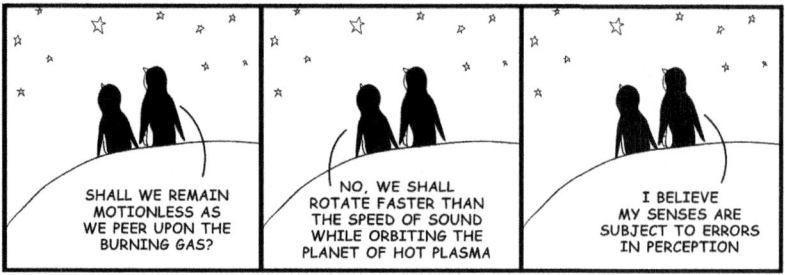

While we've focused a lot on how to see things from a neurotypical point of view, your ability to look at things differently is also your greatest strength. One of the first times I realized this was working with a young student on a school robotics project.

All the children in the class were given a box of identical supplies and were asked to build a robot. The child I was working with, "Peter," had been diagnosed with autism and had no previous building experience. Each child worked alone, and as the robots took form it soon became noticeable that there were nineteen robots with a horizontal shape and then Peter's that was vertical. His robot stuck out awkwardly from the crowd with the top of it well above the line of all the rest. Some of the children snickered with a "Peter's done it wrong again" look, but, absorbed in the project, he didn't notice and just kept building.

The robots were then brought together to perform simple tasks such as speeding across the room and touching objects. The children talked excitedly about their designs, gave compliments, and shared ideas. No one asked Peter about his. Next, the robots had to do a series of more complicated tasks involving reaching for items on a board. The first robot stretched up its arm but was too low to the ground to touch any of the objects. The next robot had the same problem and the next. The children's faces saddened as they all realized their robots' limitations. Then Peter's robot came up, the tall out-of-place creation. It stretched up its arm high and easily grabbed the objects.

Celebrate Your Differences

The class fell silent, as they all looked at his robot, looked at all the others, and mutters of "wow" were heard.

This natural ability to see things from a different perspective, and to create something new, is one of the great strengths of being on the spectrum. Albert Einstein's thinking about energy and mass radically changed science, and Elon Musk's engineering innovations transported ordinary people into space.

This same wonderful strength of being different is present in all the people I work with. It can be in the form of a question that others don't usually ask, in the perspective of a drawing, or in noticing something that is out of place. It might be in the development of a new product, an unusual approach to a problem, an original musical score, or a unique idea for fiction. It is your very ability to not think like others that is often at the foundation of your success.

USE YOUR TALENTS IN YOUR AREA OF INFLUENCE

I want to work with companies that make a demonstrable improvement in the world.

The key to using your talents is to start where you can, even if it means starting small. For many, this will be at a local level. Some of the parents that I have worked with who have lower-functioning children have told me how this is particularly challenging. It can be hard to focus on their child's strengths, to look at his potential, or envision how their child can find work. But everyone can make an impact. It might be noticing the missed crumbs on the lunch table and carefully wiping them up or offering a smile for others when they enter a room. There have been many times when I've seen how the development of such seemingly small skills bring pride and joy. Everyone has value.

For others, using talents in your area of influence can mean experimenting with ideas and taking the first steps to put your work into the world. Alfred Hitchcock, the famous director who also had autism characteristics, began by illustrating title cards for silent films. Susan Boyle sang in school productions.

Both were absorbed in their passions and interests and tried to do things their own way. They avoided the temptation to hold onto their skills until they got a "big break," but instead they used their gifts whenever they could.

Share through the internet, school, community centers, churches, libraries, universities, or with neighbors and friends. Become known in your community for what you are great at. Become the person to go to for your area of expertise. Build your skills. Develop your ideas. And then if a big break comes—celebrate.

HIGHLIGHT WHAT YOU CAN DO AND ADMIT WHAT YOU CAN'T

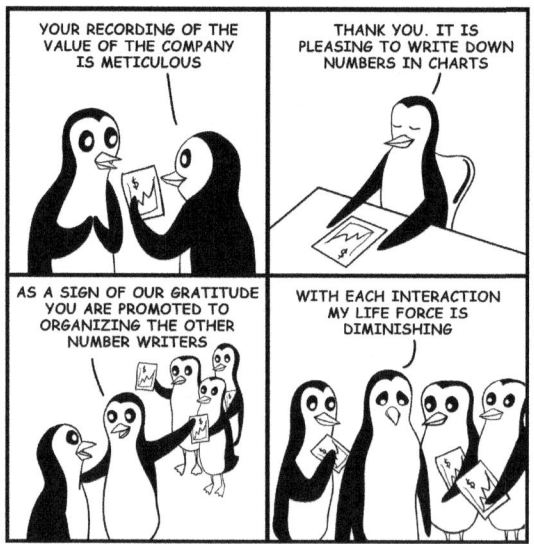

When working with clients, they will sometimes ask me if I can give them an IQ assessment or an achievement test. We usually have a good therapeutic rapport after a few sessions, and it's natural for them to believe that if I can help in one area I can also help in another. I used to do these types of assessments, but I quickly realized that I wasn't talented at analyzing the math and writing the long report. There was a time when I thought that I should be good at it. The thinking was, "If I'm good at helping people on the spectrum, then I should be good at IQ assessments." It was completely illogical, but it was there.

I see the same illogical thinking in many of my clients:

> "If I'm good at running small networks, I should be good at larger ones."
>
> "They say I'm one of the best teachers in the math department, so I'll accept the position for department chair."
>
> "As I'm a great graphic designer, I'll start an advertising agency."
>
> "I know how to run research projects, so I'll write grants for the university."
>
> "My investment figures are the highest, so I need to accept the manager position."

People will notice when your skills are high in a particular area. They will see your passion and creative thinking, but they may not fully understand what your specific skills are. Being a good graphic designer takes creativity and visual thinking. Running an advertising agency needs organization, social skills, and financial planning. The two skill sets are completely different. Just because you are good in the one area does not mean you will be good in the other. The same is true of working with figures in your head as an investment broker and managing a team of people. One job is solitary and mathematical, the other is social and verbal.

It's not that you should never try expanding your responsibilities, but when you do, be aware that you are moving into a new area. Carefully analyze what skills are needed for the position and if you are a good match.

Admitting your weaknesses can also be key in helping others to see your strengths. If you're at an interview for a computer position and you've worked on your social skills as much as you can, but it's still a challenge, then mention it to the interviewer. She can probably see it anyway, and it may be distracting her. It's much better if you address it directly and be proud of it. Your brain doesn't work like everyone else, and that's the very reason you're one of the best at what you do and why she should hire you. It's also the reason why you won't be a threat to her job. You're not so good with people.

"As you can see from my resume, I've fixed numerous networks. I'm good at going in, identifying the problem, and solving it. My mind has always had a gift for coding and math." (The interviewer is now starting to get interested in you. She can see you look different, and you're telling her you have a gift in a specific area). You pause, then say, "But I'm not good at organizing office social events, and I'm not made for managing teams. But if you need someone to fix your computers, that's me."

CELEBRATE THE DIAGNOSIS

Before I was diagnosed, I felt like I was separated from the world, like I didn't belong. Afterwards I felt the same way, but I knew I wasn't alone.

Families ask me if they should tell their child about his or her autism diagnosis. They are often afraid the diagnosis will become a burden and that their child will feel bad about themselves or give up trying. These can be valid concerns, especially if the diagnosis is given in a setting that has negative connotations. I've seen difficulties in children who learned about their diagnoses from overhearing a parent talk on the phone to the school ("It must be bad if the school called"). Others have struggled because they saw their parent crying, or they were called a name by a peer.

But as a parent, you can control how the diagnosis is given. You can set the mood and tone. Over the years, I've developed a standard way of informing a client of his or her diagnosis called, "The Mind Quest." It celebrates strengths and challenges, normalizes differences, and forms an attitude about autism that is both positive and realistic. In the example below of a child named Jenna, I'm using language that would be appropriate for her age. But the concepts work just as well with adults when adapted.

THE MIND QUEST

For this activity I like to prepare the client the week before by pointing out a strength that she has and introducing the concept of both strengths and challenges. "You're such a good artist. I love all the detail you put into the face. You have an amazing mind for remembering what things look like. I wish I had that; I'm not so good at art." Then I'll share how excited I am because in the next session we will play The Mind Quest and find out what types of minds everyone has. A child's interest can be quickly captured with comments such as, "I wonder what kind of mind your mom and dad have."

For the session, everyone in the family is given a clipboard, paper, and pencil. They draw a line down the center and put a - sign on the left and a + sign on the right, so that they have two separate columns for their strengths and challenges. I always have my own sheet and fully participate in the process as I lead it. This sends a strong message that we all have different types of minds.

As a group, we will discuss our strengths and challenges, writing them down on our sheets (younger children can draw pictures). My goal is to have the family and child be involved as much as possible. Several questions can help with this process such as:

"I wonder what Daddy's strength is. What's he good at?"

"I'm terrible at ...... How's everyone else at that?"

"What else would be on your + side?"

"I'm thinking about how good you are at fixing phones. Now what would that skill be called?"

If the client analyzes her ability in an area incorrectly, then I'll gently correct her. "Jenna, I remember you telling me it was hard to talk to people and make friends. Maybe talking to people should go on your challenges side."

Because I want the client to form a realistic understanding of what it means to have a mind on the spectrum, I'll be sure to address the key areas of social interactions, communication, cognitive, and sensorimotor. (For a reminder on what these areas include, please review Chapter 4.) I'll also teach the names of different skills such as visual processing or auditory memory.

Once the lists are complete, we will take turns exploring them. I usually start, holding up my sheet so that everyone can see it, as I read out my strengths and challenges. Because I usually have performing in front of very large crowds on my challenges side, I'll say, "I know what kind of mind I have. I have a shy mind." I'll then write the word "shy" at the bottom and take a book about shyness down from the shelf, showing that there are books about my type of mind.

Continuing around the group, we give a name to everyone's mind, either using one word or a combination of words. Some of the more common words I've used include ADHD, ADD, Asperger's, autism, extrovert, introvert, social, shy, creative, energetic, mathematical, engineering, language, dancer, and builder. Although the focus of the session is the person on the spectrum, I'll try to capture a true description of everyone in the room and show a copy of an applicable book where I have one.

For the person on the spectrum, I'll review her strengths and challenges, spending some extra time on the unique and exciting part of her strengths. Then I'll say, "I know what type of mind you have. You have an autism type of mind." I'll help her to make sense of any of her challenges through the framework of the autism. "It makes perfect sense that ... is hard for you. This is something that can be difficult for people with an autism type of mind."

I keep some printouts in my office of famous autistic people and will show these along with a copy of a book about autism. It's very important to include information about autism being a spectrum and what this might look like for different people. If I am using the word "Asperger's," I will explain that this is also called "autism." At the end of the session, I give the person a homework assignment to research famous people with autism and that we can talk about it the next time we meet.

Occasionally, after learning about her diagnosis, a child will try to get out of an activity because of being on the spectrum. Her logic usually follows something like, "Well, because of my autism I'm not good at being with people, so I shouldn't have to go to the birthday party."

As the parent, this can easily be addressed by telling her that you understand how she feels, and she is right that being with people is on her list of challenges.

Because it's something that she's not so good at, she really needs more practice than everyone else. She should be going to twice as many birthday parties, so she can get better at it. If you can, give an example from your own life of something you were not good at and had to practice more than others to become skilled.

CELEBRATE THROUGH PLAY

I really crave deep conversation about the things that I am interested in.

Play is important, especially when you are constantly being asked to adapt to a world that is not set up for you. The world of play, no matter what age you are, offers a space where you can use your imagination in any way you choose, where you set the stage and decide the outcomes. In the world of play, things are smaller, more manageable, and under your control.

If you are an adult on the spectrum, do not ignore your time to play. It could be role-playing games, science fiction, board games, puzzles, computer games, film, or TV. You might like to build, bird watch, bug watch, cook, or play chess. It doesn't matter what you are doing, just so long as you are having some fun doing it. Through play you will find others with similar interests, where you can have long and in-depth conversations about the things you love. Everyone needs such a space.

If you have a child on the spectrum, then your time to play with your child can be a time to just appreciate who he is, to pour into him your unconditional love. No expectations. No demands. No trying to get him to do it right. Just, "It's me here wanting to play with you." If you can, think back to your own childhood and try to imagine how it would have felt if one of your parents had come up to you every day and said, "Let's play." How would it have changed who you are today? How would it have affected the relationship you had with that parent?

With a younger child, play might be sitting on the floor building with blocks or lining up cars. With older children, it can be engaging in their area of interest. They might want to show you collections they have or play musical pieces. You don't need to spend a lengthy amount of time playing each day to make an impact. A few minutes every day has a positive effect. It's like putting money into the bank of the relationship, so that when you want to make a withdrawal, you can. Through play, children can become less oppositional, more connected, more confident, and verbal. I'll usually tell parents just to try it, and then see what changes they notice. Sometimes it's an extra hug, more smiles, or a greater willingness to talk. When planning your play time with your child:

- Set a goal of 15 minutes play time each day.
- Find a name for the play time such as "fun time," "game time," or "relax time." This will help your child learn that certain rules apply to this time that don't apply elsewhere.
- Tell your child that you want to have some fun time with her, and let her choose the activity.

While any type of play with your child is valuable, I've listed some guidelines for play that will help make it a therapeutic time for your child. The guidelines draw from Parent-Child Interaction Therapy and the work of Dr. Stanley Greenspan. These guidelines can be used by family, friends, teachers, or therapists. You can copy the list and have it in front of you as you play or try to practice one quality each play session. Just know that these concepts look much easier on paper than they are in practice. I still struggle with not asking indirect questions. So be gentle with yourself, have fun, and spend some time celebrating your child.

- Follow the child's lead.
    Your child will choose what he wants to play, and you will be following his lead. Pick a similar toy to the one he has chosen to

play with and imitate what he does. If he is lining up cars, you line up your cars. If she is scribbling on paper, you scribble too. If your child is older and doing something you can't do, such as playing the piano, then you can sit next to her and listen.

When you are following your child's lead, you will want to avoid giving directions, as this takes the lead away from the child. Examples of directions include, "Let's put the house here," "Why don't we stack the blocks?" "Please give me the crayon," or "Don't you think you should change the key of this song?"

When following his lead, always stay one step behind your child's level of skills. Your line of cars is not quite as straight or as long. Your pile of blocks is not as tall. Resist the temptation to solve problems for your child as he plays. For example, if he is trying to figure out how to build a bridge, don't step in and do it for him. Allow him to find his own solutions, even if this means he throws the blocks on the floor and moves on to something else.

- Vocalize the child's actions and words:

    Vocalizing your child's actions is a key element of play time. Pay attention to what she is doing, and then describe it out loud, keeping your tone of voice full of energy and enthusiasm. For example, "You're lining up all the cars." "You're going to play a song."

    Repeating what she is saying is also an essential element. If your child says, "I drew a zoo," you can say, "You drew a zoo." Vocalizing words and actions will help your child to organize her thoughts and language and shows that you're paying close attention. Children quickly will come to understand that their words are important.

- Praise often:

    Give your child plenty of genuine, specific praise. Be sure the praise is specific and tells the child exactly what you like. "It's amazing how you've memorized this whole musical score" is specific. "Well done" is not.

No matter what the situation, you can always find some things that are worthy of praise. Even a child who is having a tantrum and crying must break for a second to take a breath, giving you the opportunity to say, "Good taking a breath." As you choose different things to praise, be aware that behaviors that are praised are more likely to occur in the future.

- Avoid questions and interruptions.

   Parents ask their children questions all the time. While this is a very natural part of conversation, you will want to avoid asking questions during this play time as it takes the lead away from the child. Be careful of indirect questions such as, "That was good wasn't it?" or "Could you put this over here?"

   You will also want to avoid interruptions. Turn your phone, television, and computer off. Put your books and work away. For those parents who have more than one child, take turns playing with each child. This can be done on the same day, on different days, or by rotating between parents. When one child interrupts you while playing with another, let him know that you would love to play with him, but it is not his turn, and you will play with him later. Both children will learn the importance of boundaries and keeping commitments with others.

DO THE PENGUIN SHUFFLE

Life is full of challenges, some we can see on the horizon, and others sneak up on us. They can knock us off balance and leave us feeling vulnerable and unable to cope.

In the movie March of the Penguins (2005), there's a scene where the penguins settle down for the arctic winter. The temperature is 80 degrees below

Celebrate Your Differences

zero, and the winds are up to 100 miles an hour. Any one penguin standing alone against these forces won't survive, so they huddle together to brace the elements. Those on the outside of the group receive the worst of the storm, while those closest to the center are the most protected and feel the warmth of the other penguins. Each penguin takes turns, moving from the outside to the center and back again. This constant moving between outside and inside I call the "Penguin Shuffle."

We too will have seasons in our lives when storms come at us, and our best chance of survival will be to allow ourselves to be supported and surrounded by others. Our community of family, friends, organizations, and professionals can stand in the gaps, protecting us from the challenges we face. At other times we may be in a position of strength, and we can shuffle from the center to the outside where we can offer help and support to those around us.

Some of you have been standing in one position for too long; you might find it hard to move from the outside and accept help from others, or you might be stuck in the center not realizing that if you shuffle to the outside you have something important to give. I want you to know that when we remember to do the penguin shuffle, we all stand protected against the harshest of seasons.

THE FINAL RULE

I would like to leave you with a final rule. It is, without doubt, my favorite rule in the book and is at the heart of my work as a psychologist. Understanding who you are, educating others about how your mind works, celebrating your strengths, and learning to navigate the world around you will lead you to this rule. I want you to always remember that this rule is both relevant and true.

THE RULE IS:

GO OUT AND GIVE YOUR GIFTS TO THE WORLD, FOR YOU ARE BEAUTIFULLY AND WONDERFULLY MADE

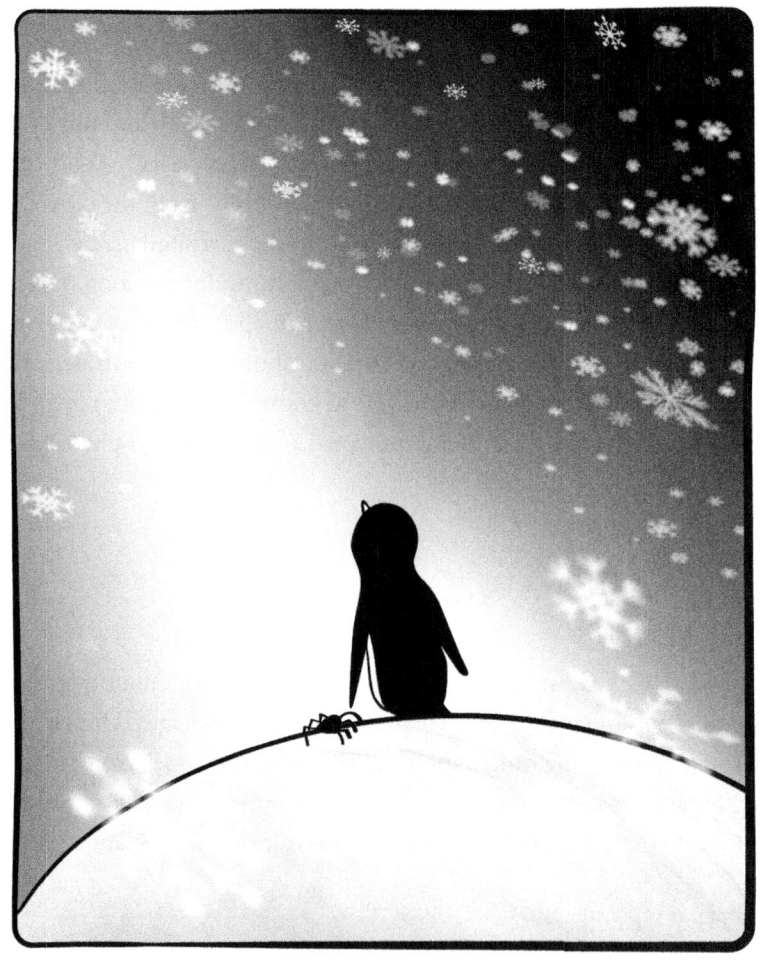

CHAPTER 6

The Rules Checklist

All the rules covered in this book are listed below. Use the rules checklist to mark off the ones you have learned or pick 3-5 goals that you want to learn first. If you are working with a child, it will be important to prioritize goals so that teachers, friends, and family will know which rules to focus on.

Preliminary Rules

- ☐ Being different is not the same as being wrong (page 13).
- ☐ Most social rules are unwritten (page 14).
- ☐ If you break an unwritten social rule, people will become angry or anxious and make a judgment about you which is usually negative and wrong (page 15).
- ☐ The typical person navigating social rules is like a bat navigating with echolocation (page 16).
- ☐ People on the spectrum have a different social radar (page 20).

AUTISM RULES

Consciously Learn The Unwritten Rules

Hygiene
- ☐ Take a shower and wash your hair every day (page 24).
- ☐ Use deodorant at least once a day (page 24).
- ☐ Keep your nails cut and clean (page 24).
- ☐ Don't wear the same clothes two days in a row (page 24).

Communication
- ☐ When talking to another person, spend more time talking about that person's interests than yours (page 25).
- ☐ Be aware that the majority of conversations are very superficial (page 25).
- ☐ Develop an index card in your mind for each person you interact with on a regular basis (page 26).
- ☐ Use the 5Ws (page 27).
- ☐ Combine the 5Ws with your index card (page 28).
- ☐ It's usually more important to be kind than to be right (page 29).
- ☐ There is a cost to free speech (page 32).

Honesty
- ☐ People want honesty, but they also don't want to be hurt emotionally (page 33).
- ☐ Answers that do not hurt a person should always be given honestly (page 35).
- ☐ Answers that will hurt the person, but are important for the person to know, should be given with (gentle) honesty (page 35).
- ☐ Answers that will hurt the person, and are not important for the person to know, should be given to meet the person's current need (page 37).

Caring For Others
- ☐ Practice cognitive caring (page 40).
- ☐ Arrive at a party 10 minutes after the given time (page 41).
- ☐ Just because hosts are being nice to you does not mean that they want you to stay (page 41).

- ☐ It's time to leave a party or event when around 50% of the guests have left (page 42).
- ☐ Never tell a child that Santa, the Easter Bunny, or the tooth fairy aren't real. Always discuss it with your partner before telling your own child (page 42).
- ☐ When you buy a present, be sure you are buying something the other person will want, rather than something you want (page 43).
- ☐ Do one kind act for a family member each day (page 43).

Boundaries

- ☐ It's okay to say no (page 45).
- ☐ If you're not in law enforcement, don't police others (page 46).
- ☐ Faith does not have to be based on feelings (page 47).
- ☐ People will respect you more if they can't take advantage of you (page 47).
- ☐ Use social stories for children (page 48).

Strengthen Your Social Radar

- ☐ It's hard for you to know what your radar is not picking up (page 56).
- ☐ Choose a social guide for your radar (page 57).
- ☐ Social radars are mainly visual (page 59).
- ☐ Learn from those who have gone before you (page 63).
- ☐ Turn the background volume down (page 64).
- ☐ Develop a sensory diet (page 67).
- ☐ Turn the anxiety down by learning what to do (page 70).
- ☐ When anxious, step 1 is to rate your anxiety (page 72).
- ☐ When anxious, step 2 is to understand fight, flight, freeze (page 74).
- ☐ When anxious, step 3 is to face the anxiety (page 76).
- ☐ When anxious, step 4 is to reduce the anxiety (page 79).
- ☐ Reduce anxiety in step 4 by breathing diaphragmatically (page 80).
- ☐ Reduce anxiety in step 4 by rewiring your brain's circuits (page 82).
- ☐ Reduce anxiety in step 4 with exercise (page 87).

- ☐ Reduce anxiety in step 4 by challenging irrational fears (page 88).
- ☐ Reduce anxiety in step 4 with progressive muscle relaxation (page 92).
- ☐ Reduce anxiety in step 4 by going back to your senses (page 94).
- ☐ Turn the anxiety down by learning what not to do (page 95).
- ☐ Develop an emergency exit plan (page 97).
- ☐ Some maps can get you lost (page 101).
- ☐ Remember to ask yourself, "What are their feelings up to?" (page 104).
- ☐ First easy, then difficult (page 105).
- ☐ Don't forget the happy ending (page 107).

Educate Others About How Your Mind Works

- ☐ It's important to explain your differences to others (page 110).
- ☐ Identify the traits of your spectrum mind (page 111).

Celebrate Your Differences And If People Don't Like It, Too Bad For Them

- ☐ You're in good company (page 131).
- ☐ You can learn from success (page 140).
- ☐ Success Strategy:
- ☐ Use a language that works for you (page 145).
- ☐ Find people who believe in you (page 145).
- ☐ Fail fast. Fail often (page 146).
- ☐ Passionately embrace your interests (page 149).
- ☐ Be an independent thinker (page 150).
- ☐ Ask for support from family and friends (page 150).
- ☐ Consider employment with routine, security, and few social demands (page 151).
- ☐ Start where you can (page 155).
- ☐ Develop a community (page 156).

The Rules Checklist

- ☐ Find mentors (page 156).
- ☐ Use your determination (page 157).
- ☐ You can learn from fictional characters (page 158).
- ☐ Seeing things differently is your greatest strength (page 162).
- ☐ Use your talents in your area of influence (page 163).
- ☐ Highlight what you can do and admit what you can't (page 164).
- ☐ Celebrate the diagnosis (page 166).
- ☐ Celebrate through play (page 169).
- ☐ Do the penguin shuffle (page 172).

- ☐ THE FINAL RULE (page 173)
    Go out and give your gifts to the world, for you are beautifully and wonderfully made.

AUTISM RULES

CHAPTER 7

Resources

Below is a list of resources that for both adults and children. It includes organizations, interventions, internet sites, and publishers.

AAPC PUBLISHING
Publisher specializing in books, webinars, and resources on autism. www.aapcpublishing.com

AMERICAN ACADEMY OF CHILD AND ADOLESCENT PSYCHIATRY: AUTISM RESOURCE CENTER.
Family information, clinical resources, videos, research, training, and literature. www.aacap.org Type "Autism Resource Center" in the search bar.

AUTISM NAVIGATOR
A valuable site that shows videos of typically developing toddlers alongside videos of toddlers with autism in similar circumstances. Differences are clearly explained in areas such as communication, social interaction, interests, gestures, non-verbal behaviors, and play. www.autismnavigator.com

AUTISM NOW
Provides resources and information on services and support across the life span. Covers areas such as home, school, work, and community. www.autismnow.org

AUTISM SELF ADVOCACY NETWORK
Empowering individuals with autism to advocate for changes in systems, policies, and civil rights. Run by and for people with autism, they seek to promote a culture of inclusion and respect for all. www.autisticadvocacy.org

AUTISM SOCIETY
This is a national society dedicated to advocacy, research, and support. www.autism-society.org

AUTISM SPECTRUM NEWS
Publication for the autism community with articles on a range of topics such as transition to adulthood and autism and women. www.mhnews-autism.org

CENTER FOR PARENT INFORMATION AND RESOURCES
Offers support, training, and information about services in your state from birth to age 26. This includes areas such as early intervention, school services, therapy, policies, transportation, employment, and independent living. www.parentcenterhub.org

CLINICAL STUDIES DATABASE
An international database of public and privately-supported ongoing and completed clinical studies. You can search by diagnosis and topic. www.clinicaltrials.gov

CRISIS TEXT LINE

Free mental health support via text. Always open and very helpful for those who would rather not speak on the phone. A live, trained crisis counselor receives the text and responds, helping you move out of a hot moment. Their counselors work with a variety of crisis situations including school stress, anxiety, depression, emotional abuse, and suicide. www.crisistextline.org

EARLY INTERVENTION

For children from birth to age 3. Provides services including speech, occupational, nutritional, and psychological. Each state runs their own program, which is often free of charge or on a sliding scale based on income. Contact your pediatrician or pediatrics department at your local hospital. You can also find your local program by visiting www.cdc.gov/ncbddd/actearly/parents/states.html

EASTERSEALS

Interventions for preschoolers, school-aged children, and adults. Programs include child care, early intervention, social integration, play, Applied Behavioral Analysis, outpatient therapy, school to work transition programs, job training, residential services, and independence training. www.easterseals.com/our-programs/autism-services/

EDUCATIONAL SERVICES

For ages 3 to 21. Services are provided through the department of special education and can include an Individualized Education Plan (IEP) or a 504 Plan. A written request for eligibility can be made by a parent, teacher, or school personnel. www.autism-society.org Type "IEP" in the search bar.

EXCEPTIONAL MINDS

A studio and academy that provides training for people on the autism spectrum for work in animation and the digital arts. www.exceptionalmindsstudio.org

FIRST WORDS PROJECT
Provides tools to support early learning and the development of language from birth to 24 months. Features hundreds of video clips to learn key social communication milestones and how you can support your child's development. Areas include play, emotional regulation, social interaction, and self-directed learning. Also includes a tool for charting your child's social communication growth. www.babynavigator.com

FLOORTIME
Created by Dr. Stanley Greenspan and his colleagues, Floortime is a relationship-based intervention that focuses on development and playful interaction. The emphasis is on engaging with your child in a setting such as your home. The DIRFloortime site has information, courses, consultations, and conferences. www.icdl.com

FUTURE HORIZONS
Specializes in books on autism spectrum disorders. www.fhautism.com

GOT TRANSITION
Helps with planning, transfer, and integration into adult-centered health care. Under the resources and research for special populations, you will find specific information for people with autism. www.gottransition.org

GRANDPARENT AUTISM NETWORK
Informs grandparents about autism and the medical, educational, legal, and social issues that affect their families. There are social and advocacy events for grandparents and grandchildren. www.ganinfo.org

HEALTH INSURANCE
I've included this on the list as a reminder that health insurance can provide many services including individual, family, speech, and occupational therapy. Although you may be receiving some of these services through the school, supplementing them with private practitioners gives an additional

perspective and help across the lifespan. Call your insurance company and ask about services for autism (Diagnosis code F84.0).

JESSICA KINGSLEY PUBLISHERS
Publishes a wide range of books focusing on autism spectrum disorders. www.jkp.com

LEARN HOW TO BECOME
Career guidance and support with information on a variety of careers, online education, interview and resume advice, and other resources. www.learnhowtobecome.org

MEDICAID WAIVER
Provides home and community services such as therapy, social groups, respite, residential, and case management. The Medicaid Waiver site gives information on the specific services in each of the states. www.medicaidwaiver.org/

NATIONAL DISABILITIES RIGHTS NETWORK (NDRN)
For protection and advocacy services in your state. www.ndrn.org

ORGANIZATION FOR AUTISM RESEARCH (OAR)
Focuses on research that enhances the day-to-day quality of life of individuals with autism. Areas supported include education, communication, self-care, social skills, employment, behavior, and adult and community living. You can download several free guidebooks on topics such as safety, navigating the special education system, life as a sibling, and assessment. www.researchautism.org

REDDIT
Several of my clients have found reddit a very helpful place to chat with people on the spectrum and with people who know someone with autism. You will find postings that are humorous, give practical advice, share experiences, ask questions, and offer support. You will

also find several subgroups, such as girls with autism. As with any site where there are unknown visitors, children will need to be supervised. www.reddit.com/r/autism

SIBLING SUPPORT PROJECT
Provides help for siblings of people with health, developmental, and mental health concerns. The program has books, articles, online groups, and workshops. It can also help you set up a sibling support group in your local community. www.siblingsupport.org

SPECIAL NEEDS ALLIANCE
National organization that can help you find a nearby attorney dedicated to the practice of disability and public benefits law. Their attorneys have an average of 18 years of relevant experience, and are allowed to join by invitation only. There is also a newsletter and blog. www.specialneedsalliance.org

SPECIAL OLYMPICS
Year-round sports training and athletic competition for people with intellectual disabilities, helping them discover strengths, skills, and success. It also develops connections for their friends and families. www.specialolympics.org

SUPPLEMENTAL SECURITY INCOME (SSI)
Supplemental income for those who are considered disabled and in need of extra income. Contact the Social Security Administration www.ssa.gov

THE ART OF AUTISM
Supports artists, musicians, and creative writers on the autism spectrum. There are forums for displaying and promoting art, blogs, and poetry. The site also has relevant articles and listings of other artistic organizations for artists with autism. www.the-art-of-autism.com

U.S. DEPARTMENT OF HEALTH AND HUMAN SERVICES
General information, diagnosis, resources, treatment, publications, and research. www.hhs.gov

VOCATIONAL REHABILITATION
Every state has a vocational rehabilitation (VR) agency that can help with employment counseling, job training, placement and support. Your state agency will assess eligibility and develop an individualized plan depending on your needs. rsa.ed.gov/

ZERO TO THREE
Ensures that babies and toddlers get a strong start in life by supporting families, policymakers, and professionals. Provides resources, knowledge, fellowships, virtual events, guides, podcasts, newsletters, and a bookstore. www.zerotothree.org

AUTISM RULES

REFERENCES

Access. "The Good Doctor Star Freddie Highmore on Responsibility of Showing Autism Authentically." YouTube, Oct. 2017, www.youtube.com/watch?v=pVe33jbLRO0.

Aykroyd, Dan. "The Big Interview with Dan Rather – Dan Aykroyd." AXS TV, Nov. 2018, www.axs.tv/channel/the-big-interview-with-dan-rather-season-6/video/dan-aykroyd/.

Aykroyd, Peter, and Angela Narth. A History of Ghosts: The True Story of Séances, Mediums, Ghosts and Ghostbusters. Rodale Books, 2009.

BBC. "Climate Change: Greta Thunberg School Strikes Began a Year Ago." Newsround, Aug. 2019, www.bbc.co.uk/newsround/49405357.

Berger, Eric. Liftoff: Elon Musk and the Desperate Early Days that Launched SpaceX. William Morrow an imprint of HarperCollins, 2021.

Boyle, Susan. The Woman I was Born to Be: My Story. Atria Books, 2010.

Brian, Denis. Einstein: A Life. 1st ed., John Wiley & Sons, 1997.

Brian Linehan's City Lights. "Anthony Hopkins Interview 1978." YouTube, Sept. 2015, www.youtube.com/watch?v=pmpps5dL6tc.

Britain's Got Talent. "Susan Boyle's first audition – 'I dreamed a dream,'" YouTube, Mar. 2019, www.youtube.com/watch?v=yE1Lxw5ZyXk.

Calaprice, Alice. Dear Professor Einstein: Albert Einstein's Letters to and From Children. 1st ed., Prometheus Books, 2002.

Chalakoski, Martin. "Sir Anthony Hopkins won the Oscar for role of psychopath Hannibal Lecter with only 16 minutes of screen time and an unblinking stare..." The Vintage News, Nov. 2017, www.thevintagenews.com/2017/11/29/anthony-hopkins/.

Condivi, Ascanio. The Life of Michelangelo. Translated by Charles Holroyd, Pallas Athene, 2007.

Cooper-White, Macrina. "Temple Grandin on the Secret to Success for Kids with Autism." Huffpost, Aug. 2014, www.huffingtonpost.com/2014/08/29/temple-grandin-interview-huffpost_n_5676121.html.

Deveney, Catherine. "Susan Boyle: My Relief at Discovering that I Have Asperger's." The Guardian, 7 Dec. 2013, www.theguardian.com/music/2013/dec/08/susan-boyle-autism.

Diament, Michelle. "Actors with Autism Join Netflix Series 'Atypical.'" Disability Scoop, Sept. 2018, www.disabilityscoop.com/2018/09/11/actors-autism-netflix-atypical/25474/.

Dr. Infographics. "Elon Musk 'I don't give a damn about your degree.'" YouTube, Feb. 2018, www.youtube.com/watch?v=CQbKctnnA-Y.

Einstein, Albert. Autobiographical Notes. Translated and edited by Paul Arthur Schilpp, Open Court, 1999.

Einstein, Albert. The Collected Papers of Albert Einstein. Princeton University Press. einsteinpapers.press.princeton.edu.

Einstein, Albert. The Ultimate Quotable Einstein. Collected and edited by Alice Calaprice, Princeton University Press, 2013.

Einstein, Albert. The World as I See It. Createspace, 2014.

Einstein, Albert, and Mileva Maric. Albert Einstein / Mileva Maric: The Love Letters, edited by Jurgen Renn and Robert Schulmann. Translated by Shawn Smith, Princeton University Press, 2000.

Ewing, Sarah. "'I have Asperger's – one of my symptoms included being obsessed with ghosts': Under the microscope with Dan Aykroyd." The Daily Mail, Dec. 2013, www.dailymail.co.uk/health/article-2521032/Dan-Aykroyd-I-Aspergers-symptoms-included-obsessed-ghosts.html.

Fossey, Dian. Gorillas in the Mist. Mariner Books, 2000.

References

Fossey, Dian. "Years with the Mountain Gorilla, 1973. The Leakey Foundation." YouTube, Feb. 2019. www.youtube.com/watch?v=MVtlTFas5w4

Gannon, Louis. "From the Valleys . . . To Transformers?" Pressreader, June 2017.

Goodman, Amy. "School Strike for Climate: Meet 15-Year-Old Activist Greta Thunberg, Who Inspired a Global Movement." Democracy Now, Dec. 2018.www.democracynow.org/2018/12/11/meet_the_15_year_old_swedish.

Grandin, Temple. "Temple Grandin Interview – Part 1. Whitworth University." YouTube, Aug. 2016. www.youtube.com/watch?v=31iRJeRpA3w.

Grandin, Temple. Thinking in Pictures: My Life with Autism. Vintage, 2006.

Greenspan, Stanley, and Serena Wieder. Engaging Autism. Using the Floortime Approach to Help Children Relate, Communicate, and Think. Da Capo Lifelong Books. 2006

Greenstreet, Rosanna. "Q & A: Susan Boyle." The Guardian, 13 Dec. 2014, www.theguardian.com/lifeandstyle/2014/dec/13/susan-boyle-interview.

Hopkins, Anthony. "The Anthony Hopkins LEAP Seminar." YouTube, July 2018, www.youtube.com/watch?v=2t-dqDiXQ2k.

Hopkins, Anthony. "If You Only Knew: Anthony Hopkins, Larry King Now." YouTube, May 2016, www.youtube.com/watch?v=-oT63andb1k.

Isaacson, Walter. Einstein: His life and Universe. Paperback ed., Simon & Schuster, 2017.

Jarmachi. "Satoshi Tajiri's Game Design Lessons." YouTube, March. 2020, https://www.youtube.com/watch?v=N_G7qXd_Pmk&t=31s.

Jimmy Kimmel Live. "Anthony Hopkins Shares an Important Life Lesson." YouTube, June 2017, www.youtube.com/watch?v=p3Un_eyuyOI.

Johnston, Jenny. "The truth about my Asperger's: Susan Boyle reveals just how difficult it is living with a condition that makes her behaviour so very unpredictable." The Daily Mail, Nov. 2014. www.dailymail.co.uk/femail/article-2828626/The-truth-Asperger-s-Susan-Boyle-reveals-just-difficult-living-condition-makes-behaviour-unpredictable.html.

Jordan, Mary. "Along with 'Talent,' Susan Boyle Shows the World Her Temper, Too." The Washington Post, 29 May 2009, www.washingtonpost.com/wp- dyn/content/article/2009/05/28/ AR2009052803745.html.

March of the Penguins. Dir. by Luc Jacquet. Buena Vista International, 2005.

McNeil, Cheryl, and Toni Hembree-Kigin. Parent-Child Interaction Therapy. Springer, 2010.

Montgomery, Alice. Susan Boyle: Dreams Can Come True. The Overlook Press, 2010.

Musk, Maye. A Woman Makes a Plan: Advice for a Lifetime of Adventure, Beauty, and Success. Penguin Life, 2020.

Neffe, Jurgen. Einstein: A Biography. Translated by Shelley Frisch. 1st ed., Farrar, Straus and Giroux, 2007.

NorCalKay. "Susan Boyle Intimately Reflects on Past and Present with Fern Britton." YouTube, 1 Dec. 2013, www.youtube.com/watch?v=uPxPMOVnujo&t=1223s.

NorCalKay. "Susan Boyle. There's Something About Susan. Coping with Asperger's in 1st-Ever Concert." YouTube, 12 Dec. 2013, www.youtube.com/watch?v=g8oTvPMRNIg.

Parker, Barry. Einstein: The Passions of a Scientist. 1st ed., Prometheus Books, 2003.

"2004 PETA Proggy Award: Visionary Winner: Temple Grandin." Abolitionist Approach, www.abolitionistapproach.com/media/links/p1511/2004peta.pdf. Accessed Aug. 2020.

Pokemon the Movie: Diancie and the Cocoon of Destruction. Dir. Kunihiko Yuyama. Toho, 2014.

Pokemon the Movie: Hoopa and the Clash of Ages. Dir. Kunihiko Yuyama. Toho, 2015.

Polinsky, Paige V. Pokemon Designer: Satoshi Tajiri. Checkerboard Library, 2017.

Prince-Hughes, Dawn. Songs of the Gorilla Nation: My Journey Through Autism. Broadway Books, 2005.

References

Prince-Hughes, Dawn. "Through the Looking Glass." National Public Radio, Snap Judgement. 27 Feb. 2015, www.npr.org/2015/02/27/389489102/through-the-looking-glass.

Sesame Street. "Julia and Grover search for patterns." YouTube, Apr. 2018, www.youtube.com/watch?v=Jl7EwPp6HQ0.

60 Minutes. "2012: SpaceX: Elon Musk's race to space." YouTube, Dec. 2018, www.youtube.com/watch?v=23GzpbNUyI4.

Strauss, Neil. "Elon Musk: The Architect of Tomorrow." Rolling Stone, no. 1301, 15 November 2017, www.rollingstone.com/culture/culture-features/elon-musk-the-architect-of-tomorrow 120850/.

Tajiri, Satoshi. "The Ultimate Game Freak." Time Magazine. 22 Nov. 1999, content.time.com/time/magazine/article/0,9171,2040095,00.html.

Temple Grandin. Dir. Mick Jackson. HBO, 2010.

Thunberg, Greta, and Svante Thunberg, Malena Ernman, Beata Ernman. Our House is on Fire: Scenes of a Family and a Planet in Crisis. Penguin, 2020.

Today. "What to Know About Being a Good Friend to Someone with Autism, According to Sesame Street." YouTube, Apr. 2018, www.youtube.com/watch?v=sNms-nmhCEI.

Vance, Ashlee. Elon Musk: Tesla, SpaceX, and the Quest for a Fantastic Future. Ecco an imprint of HarperCollins, 2015.

INDEX

Abstract reasoning, 125
Acts of kindness, 43
Alcohol, 95-96
Alone time, 124
Anxiety, 70-100
Asking for help, 119
Aykroyd, Dan, 137

Balance, 123
Boone, Christopher, 159
Boyle, Susan, 141-146, 163

Chewing sounds, 93
Clumsy, 123
Cognitive caring, 40
Conversation, 25-28, 117-119
Copying others, learn by, 63
Criticism, accepting, 129

Darth Vader breath, 80-82
Depression, 129

Detail-oriented, 126
Diagnosis, celebrate, 166-172
Different is not wrong, 13-14
Distracted, 128-129
Drug use, 95-96

Echolocation, 16
Einstein, Albert, 147-151
Elevator experiment, 15
Empathy, 40, 113
Exit plan, 97-100
Eye contact, 59, 112

Fabric sensitivity, 122
Facial expressions, 112
Feeling different, 13, 127
Fight, flight, freeze, 74-76
Final rule, 173-174
Fossey, Dian, 133
Free speech, 32

Gardner, Sam, 161
Getting along with others, 113
Gift giving, 43
Grandin, Temple, 135-136

Handwriting, poor, 124
Honesty, 33-39, 119
Hopkins, Sir Anthony, 133-135
Hygiene, 24

Inappropriate questions, 118
Index card system, 26-28

Index

Interests, 119, 125
Irrational fears, challenge, 88-91

Julia, 158-159

Kindness, 29-31, 43-44

Language, sounds different, 118
Leaving an event, 42, 107
Lies, 33
Lights, 121
Literal, 117

Making friends, 116
Mapping, 101-103, 115
Michelangelo, 132
Mind Quest, 167-169
Monopolizing conversation, 25-28, 119
Murphy, Dr. Shaun, 160-161
Musk, Elon, 137-139

Neurotypicals, 16-17, 128

Occupational therapist, 68
On No Land, 82-86
Out of place, noticing things are, 120
Overreacting, 114

Party etiquette, 41-42
Penguin Shuffle, 172-173
Perfectionists, 128
Physical closeness, 114
Picky eater, 120

Play, 169-172
Policing others, 46
Polite conversations, 25-28
Presents, 43
Prince-Hughes, Dawn, 65-67
Progressive muscle relaxation, 92-93
Proprioception (body awareness), 65, 123
Protecting yourself, 45, 47-48,

Respect, 47-48

Santa, 42
Saying no, 45
Senses (5...4...3...2...1), 94
Sensory diet, 67-70
Sensory noise, 64-67
Smells, 123
Social anxiety, 71, 97-100
Social guide, 57-58
Social media, 32
Social radar, 20-21, 59-62
Social stories, 48-53
Sound sensitivity, 93, 121
Special events, conversations at, 28
Stimming, 123-124
Substance abuse, 95-96
Sudden changes, 116

Tajiri, Satoshi, 152-157
Talents, using your, 163-164
Thunberg, Greta, 139-140
Touch, 122

Index

Unwritten social rules, 14-16

Visual processing, 59-62, 126
Visualization technique, 78-79
Voice, sounds different, 118
Vestibular (balance), 123

Ws, the 5, 27-28
Working in groups, 113
Writing, 126

PLEASE REVIEW THIS BOOK

If you think this book will be a helpful resource for others please take a moment to review it on the site where you purchased it, mention it on your social media, and tell your friends and family!

I'd also love to hear your ideas. If you have a rule, resource, or inspirational person that you would like to be included in this book, please email it to info@drchristinele.com

By working together, we can make the world more neurodiverse friendly.

Thank you so much!
Scan code to review on Amazon

Printed in Great Britain
by Amazon